JUDE WILLHOFF

Living Well WITH CHRONIC PAIN

Living Well

With Chronic Pain

Because life won't wait...

Instead of pain controlling you, control it with lifestyle changes and the use of Medtronic Advanced Pain Therapies.

Living Well With Chronic Pain
Nonfiction

Health/Inspirational/Self-Help

Copyright 2013 by Jude Willhoff

ISBN- 978-0-9896380-7-4

Cover design by The Killion Group
Interior format by The Killion Group
http://thekilliongroupinc.com

WHAT OTHERS ARE SAYING ABOUT THIS BOOK

"The subject is a universal one and should appeal to a huge audience. Willhoff knows whereof she speaks (having suffered with chronic pain), so she hits the points any pain sufferer would want to hear, including all the attendant feelings, emotions, desperation, social/familial implications. That she found methods to live with the pain is commendable—the reader will want to relate. But she also lives beyond the pain, as do others she highlights, and that is inspiration for any pain sufferer. This book details the control of different kinds of pain and the helpful Medtronic technologies."
—*Writers Digest*

"Jude Willhoff's story is a gift of hope and inspiration to anyone suffering from chronic pain. It has the ability to pull us back from the brink of desperation and give us the strength to go on with our lives. If you don't think there is a way out— you're wrong. This book will outline a path to your new life! If your doctor doesn't have a copy of this book, get him one."
—*Capri, Failed Back Syndrome*

"The book, Living Well With Chronic Pain, adds up to a much-needed message of hope for those caught in the clutches of chronic pain."
—*Bill Radford, The Colorado Springs Gazette*

"Jude shares her personal journey through managing chronic pain with warmth and optimism. She gives the reader hope that there is life after chronic pain. With the practical advice and coping strategies included, this book is a must for chronic pain sufferers and their care givers."
—*Lisa Shetler, Massage Therapist*

"I met you briefly on Saturday at your signing at Invesco Field in Denver. You don't know, on second thought of course you do, how good it feels to meet someone who has been where I am today. I would say that I am perhaps as close to "ending it" as you can be, after 18 years of chronic pain, the last ten being the hardest. So it was truly wonderful to read your story. Just to hear that you got off all drugs and your life got better again, has given me such hope. Thank you for writing this book, thank you for renewing my hope." I took it home the day I bought it and finished it by the following evening. I am in the process of being tested to see if the Medtronic Advanced Pain Therapy will work for me.
—*Jeannie Stephens, Chronic Back Pain*

ACKNOWLEGMENTS TO

The millions of people who are coping with Chronic Pain on their own.

AND TO

Medtronic: A world leader in medical technology, pioneering pain therapies which restore health, extend life and alleviate pain.

AND A HEARTFELT THANK YOU TO

Dr. Patrick Higgins and Staff - My family physician who has gone beyond the call of duty, taking the time to get me the help I needed and encouraging me to write this book.

Dr. Kevin C. Murphy Ph.D - For helping me find myself in the middle of excruciating pain and for teaching me how to regain control of my life.

Dr. Michael Brown, Neurosurgeon - An angel in disguise with gifted hands during my spinal cord implant surgery.

Dr. John Tyler - For having the courage to work with chronic pain patients and for your encouragement in writing this book.

AND TO MY FAMILY

Robert J. Willhoff Jr.
My hero, my husband, the love of my life who
stands beside me through my trials and
tribulations.

AND TO THE REST OF MY
WONDERFUL FAMILY

Robert J. Willhoff III,
Kevin, Jessica and Natalie Willhoff
John, Aimee, Lydia and Hannah King
Robert, Jennifer, Makaela and Jayda Powilleit.
For the way you've all shown your love and support.

TABLE OF CONTENTS

* The Pikes Peak Pain Management center no longer exists.

FOREWORD BY

Dr. Kevin C. Murphy, Ph.D.

Many excellent books have been written on the devastating, life-changing effects of chronic pain. Most focus on helping individuals to better cope with the physical, emotional, social, and work-related changes that accompany long-standing pain. Such books are written by those of us who work with people in constant pain and represent an "*outsider's*" view of a person who actually has pain that does not go away.

Ms. Willhoff has written an excellent "*insider's*" account of her own chronic pain experience from injury through recovery. With great sensitivity and clarity, she takes on the extremely difficult journey of one person caught in the grip of unrelenting pain. Her honesty combined with many useful tips on how to better manage chronic pain make this book a unique contribution.

I believe her information will prove invaluable to anyone having chronic pain. *Living Well With Chronic Pain* will save sufferers a great deal of time on their own journey toward recovery. It will not only be shortened by the knowledge she shares, but also by showing those in her same situation that they are not alone in the struggle. Her clear message is one of hope and courage. If she has been brave enough to take back her own life against great odds, she suggests that so might we all. I am honored to have witnessed her changes and hope her book lightens the burden of pain sufferers everywhere.

— Kevin C. Murphy, Ph.D.

INTRODUCTION

Living Well With Chronic Pain is the story of how I regained control of my life from constant, excruciating pain. With a mixture of personal journal entries, success stories and narrative from others, I tell the story of how I moved from the diagnosis, fear, anger, denial, and confusion in my life to the acceptance and spiritual growth I needed to survive.

Without intervention from a pain management program and Medtronic Advanced Pain Therapy, I would have ended my life. Instead, I chose to empower myself with education to fight back. Pain is recognized as a major US public health problem. Various studies estimate that chronic pain affects 15 to 33% of the US population, or as many as 86 million people. In fact, chronic pain disables more people than cancer or heart disease and costs the American people more than both combined. Pain cost an estimated $70 billion a year in medical costs, lost working days, and workers' compensation.

Statistics show one out of three people will have chronic debilitating pain. Many people I talk with about this condition either have it or know of someone who is dealing with it on a daily basis.

Incurable pain wears down the body and the mind. It can lead to physical, psychological and financial meltdown. The idea of becoming a burden to loved ones and deteriorating to a point of helplessness is a person's worst nightmare, and indeed, many people who've been diagnosed with a life sentence of chronic pain have committed suicide.

I have written the book I needed to read when I was diagnosed with this condition to help other people who are struggling with chronic pain cope in a positive manner. There is no doubt in my mind that others can learn how to get control of the pain and live a productive life. This is possible through lifestyle changes and the use of Medtronic Advanced Pain Therapies described within this book.

Half of finding out what you are in life is finding out what you are not. The day I was diagnosed, I learned I wasn't invincible. The doctors finally knew what caused the pain in my lower back and down my hips and legs. I was told I have Arachnoiditis, an inflammation of the membrane covering the spinal cord, which causes severe pain by pressing on the nerve roots resulting in Chronic Pain Syndrome (CPS). There is no cure and no more denying it. I'd been sentenced to a life of constant, unrelenting pain. This was to be my future.

Later, after much soul searching and self discovery, I learned something else: *There is real help for CPS patients.* Medical technology is an amazing thing. After going through a pain management program, I knew how to live with my chronic pain in a positive, successful manner, while staying drug free. Then, in a short time, my disease progressed and the pain became more severe down my hips and legs, and once again, I was nearly unable to walk.

I was lucky. With the huge advancement in medical technology and the recommendation from Dr. Charles Ripp (an anesthesiologist specializing in pain management treatments), I found myself a candidate for Medtronic Advanced Pain Therapy Neurostimulation, using an Itrell III spinal cord implant. I had never heard of such a thing. He went on to explain that a small device would be placed in my hip and a lead wire would wind up my spine going directly into my nerves to stop the pain.

Instead of the excruciating pain I was experiencing, after the surgery I would feel electrical pulse rates. I would have a hand-held monitor which I would place over the hip implant and could control the stimulation, deciding whether to increase or decrease it, depending on my pain level.

I talked it over with my husband and decided I had to go for it. Waking up after the surgery, the first words I heard were, "Mom's bionic." I wasn't bionic, but my life had changed yet again. Something foreign had been placed in my body. I could feel the wire going up my spine and the incisions in my hip and upper spine. At first this idea was hard to grasp. It was the kind of thing I read about, saw in the movies or heard on the late news. It didn't seem real, except for the pain from the incisions and the wire going up my spine, which in reality was quite small, but felt like the transatlantic cable.

That was in 1997. Today people don't know I have chronic pain unless I tell them. I thank God everyday for Advanced Pain Therapy from Medtronic and the precision of Dr. Michael Brown's hands when he performed my surgery. This technology is a marvel.

At this time in my life I can't feel the wires and don't even know the implant is there, except when I use my small hand held monitor to increase or decrease the stimulation. Instead of pain, I feel a tingling sensation. What a wonderful invention. No more suffering. I can walk, laugh, and be almost what people call normal. A true miracle, considering where I was coming from.

This technology is a godsend for people suffering with CPS. With the knowledge I gained in the pain management program, and the help of the spinal cord implant, I can live a nearly pain-free existence. There is real help for chronic pain sufferers.

Of course, when I turn the implant off, the pain is still *with* me. That will never change. However, with the implant I control my level of pain, totally drug free.

Who would've thought I'd have a spinal cord implant? Certainly not me. After all, I was the person who never got sick or had any kind of surgery—until now. And if I can handle the idea of having wires in me and feeling pulse rates running up and down my hips and legs in place of pain, then so can you.

I consider myself extremely fortunate to be one of the few who get to live more freely with chronic pain. My advice is for anyone suffering with CPS to give yourself a chance: Go to a pain management center. Talk to a pain management doctor about this new technology. See if it can help you live a more productive life. With education and Advanced Pain Therapy from Medtronic, there is hope for us all. Life is fragile. Live it everyday to the fullest and cherish those you love. The following is my story—clawing my way out of the darkness and back into the light.

May you be blessed on your journey,
Jude Willhoff,
Author/Speaker/Survivor
www.JudeWillhoff.com

CHAPTER ONE

Character is Who You Are
When Nobody's Looking

"Although the world is full of suffering, it is also full of the overcoming of it." *- Helen Keller*

The winter weather matched my mood—bleak and dismal. I watched the freezing rain drizzle from the gray leaden sky outside my bedroom window. My life, as I had known it, had been ripped apart. I had been raised to believe the good Lord never gave us more than we could handle. Today, I questioned my faith. Where was God? Why didn't He answer my prayers? I held the bottle of narcotic pain pills in my shaking hand, thinking how easy it would be to end it all. But the thought of not being with my husband and not seeing my children grow up held me back.

Six months earlier in Las Vegas, when I'd bent over the pool table to stroke in the eight ball, a shooting pain rushed down my lower back and right leg. A hush fell over the crowd. The butterflies in the pit of my stomach turned to bat wings. The score was tied ten to ten. This was game point. If I made it, we'd be in the finals of the Billiard Congress of America Women's National Eight Ball Championship. I had trouble standing up, but the place went wild when the eight ball dropped.

Suddenly and without warning everything changed for me. I watched the rain make tracks across the window pane. Joy had left me. My team had started playing for another season without me. They were going to defend the title I helped win. All I had left were memories. I stared at the phone. It didn't ring. Most of my friends had moved on. Like the rain, a tear tracked its way down my cheek.

The pain started as a low back ache. I thought I'd pulled a muscle. When it didn't get any better I went to see my family doctor. After many tests, he told me he couldn't find what caused my constant pain and sent me to several specialists.

Time passed and within a few months I could barely walk without assistance. I was alone with my pain. Life went on around me as my friends and family moved on with their daily business. Each day I could physically feel and see myself deteriorating as I sat and faced my own mortality. This wasn't living. This was existing.

Before I took a step that would be irreversible, I put the bottle of narcotic pain pills down and picked up my personal journal and started writing. Writing was the only thing I could do to help save what was left of my sanity.

Journal Entry, November 18, 1995

At forty-five I feel old and frightened...used up. Understanding why this has happened to me is beyond my grasp. I'm living in a state of shock. I've always been a healthy, active person, and now I'm on my way to becoming totally disabled. The doctors don't know what's wrong with me. One had the nerve to tell me it was all in my head. It's not true, it's in my back, hips and legs, everywhere, but my head.

Each day is a struggle and it's harder to get around in my home. I ask myself, why is this happening to me? There are no answers. I don't want to live...not like this. My mind still works, but my body is giving up on me. With each new day the pain becomes more unbearable. I can't work or take care of my home. I feel as if I'm of no use to anyone.

Being a Christian and loving my family, I know suicide isn't the answer, but when the pain intensifies, I think about ending my life...now with dignity...before it's too late. I hurt badly and I'm fearful of what the future holds for me. God, please give me the strength to endure this pain.

The days dragged after my husband went to work and children left for school. Alone, I sat in my darkened living room with the drapes closed. After taking my narcotics, the only place I felt comfortable was in my recliner. I shouldn't say comfortable—nothing was comfortable—but at least there, the pain was bearable.

My nights consisted of tossing and turning. Muscle spasms and unrelenting pain kept me awake. What was happening to my mind and body was beyond reason. I yearned for my old life back.

Each day I sank deeper into depression. My family tried to pull me back, but I stayed out of their reach. Angry at the world for what had happened to me, I took it out on the people close to me, the people I loved. Even in my drugged haze, I knew my family loved me, but for reasons I couldn't understand, I lashed out at them. The anger ate away at my soul.

I hated what my life had become. I hated my helplessness. And I detested the narcotics, but needed to take them to get through each day. Trapped in my pain-racked body there was no way out. Not being able to work or take care of my family, I felt useless. One day merged with the next as my insides shook from the drugs. I wanted to put a stop to the madness.

Through my fogged brain I heard the phone ring. The answering machine picked up. I listened to Dr. Higgins say, "Jude, are you there?"

He knew I was home. Where else would I...could I go? I didn't go anywhere except to his office. I answered, "Hello, it's me."

"Jude, I have some news. I received the results back from the neurologist. I want you to come into the office so we can discuss your treatment."

"What is it? What's wrong with me?" *It wasn't just in my head. They had found something.*

"Hold on, we'll talk about everything when you get here. Can your husband bring you in this afternoon at about one?"

"Yes. I'll be there." Finally, they knew what caused my pain. Had God sent me a message? Maybe he hadn't forsaken me after all. This was a step toward recovery.

Later in the day Dr. Higgins dashed my glimmering hopes when he told me I had an incurable progressive disease of the spinal cord called Arachnoiditis. He said it was clumping of the nerve roots, which caused muscle spasms and persistent pain. There is no cure. The pain would be constant for the rest of my life with a symptom of my disease called Chronic Pain Syndrome. I was told I would probably be in a wheelchair in the near future. Numbed by this information, I let him make an appointment for me at a pain management center.

While waiting to hear if my health insurance would cover me, life went on and somehow I got wrapped back up into the flow. Perhaps, not a major part, but at least glad I was still with the living. Was this a quiet call for peace coming from my soul? I was lost, but knew I wanted to live.

Journal Entry, December 14, 1995
I sit in my recliner in the living room writing in my journal. Dr. Higgins must be wrong. I can't believe there's no cure. Of course, they can cure it. It isn't cancer. Surely they have a magic pill that will make it all go away.

Today he faxed my medical records and his prescription for treatment to my insurance company. I pray a lot while I wait to hear if they'll take care of my expenses to go into the pain management program. I'm afraid of what will happen to me if they turn me down. I can't afford to attend the program without their financial help. Unfortunately, working with insurance companies can be quite difficult. They are great until you need them...then all kinds of hell breaks loose.

With my medical condition being so rare, the insurance company has to call a special committee meeting to discuss my medical records in order to decide if I'll have coverage.

They'll let me know in a few weeks. Does anyone care that the pain increases on a daily basis while I wait for strangers to decide my fate? Waiting is frustrating and infuriating. I'm less important than their bottom line. Their attitude dehumanizes me.

My inability to work is causing a strain on my family. I used to work as a freelance make-up artist, doing hair, make-up, wardrobe, and special effects for movies and commercials, making good money. Without being able to pull my share of the load, things aren't getting any easier. Losing my financial independence is a scary thing.

When Dr. Higgins diagnosed me with Arachnoiditis, he told me I would qualify for Social Security disability benefits. At the time I didn't want to bother with it. I had always worked and earned an income, and I was too proud to ask for money from anyone. Now, any money coming in would help. So much for pride.

I went to the Social Security office with high hopes. Being one hundred percent disabled, with a noncurable progressive disease such as Arachnoiditis, I shouldn't have any problem qualifying for a total medical disability. They'd requested my medical records, and then—I couldn't believe it!—but I was turned down. I went back to see Dr. Higgins. He told me not to worry, to keep trying, that sometimes it takes patients three or four times before they get their benefits.

However he did recommend an attorney to take care of my case. Eventually, I would go before a judge. In time, I would get disability benefits. I'd been paying in money for many years and it didn't seem fair that the Social Security Department made it this hard to get benefits. We have health insurance, thank goodness, but everything costs so much! I continue to fight the system, but I can't help wonder if my health insurance company would pay for my one chance to live a reasonably normal life by letting me go into the pain management program.

Journal Entry, January 29, 1996

The holidays passed in a drugged blur. It's been ages since I've gone out, except to see doctors. The pain isn't going to go away. The disease exists inside my body. I'll never be the person I was. Things have changed for me and I have to face it.

I'm angry at the world for what has happened to me; at being afflicted with a disease few people have ever heard of; at having what are supposed to be the best years of my life turn into the worst; at the Social Security Administration for withholding my own money and the insurance company for treating my life so casually. And I'm angry with my family for not understanding. Rationally, I know no one can understand without experiencing chronic pain for himself, but I'm so alone. In my heart, I know I have to be strong for myself, or I'll be lost. Fear of what the future holds in store for me is very real. Can anyone help me? God knows I don't know how to help myself. They're all going on with their lives and I'm stuck in the seventh level of hell.

People I thought were my friends don't have time for me. They have fallen by the wayside and this causes another kind of pain. I quickly discover who my real friends are. They are sticking it out with me by keeping in touch. Unknown to them, these people and my family are my lifeline.

My family tried to show their love and support by caring for me even though it was hard to deal with my moodiness and pain. I knew that, yet I also knew they were going on and I couldn't help but resent them. It didn't matter that it was neither by their choice or mine. Every day reminded me they could and would function without me. Families do it every day, because they have to. Anger, frustration and helplessness ruled my life.

The narcotics kept me on an emotional roller coaster. Not taking the drugs wasn't the answer. Without them I couldn't stand the pain. I was caught in a dark, scary place. I didn't want to live being dependent on drugs and other people. And I didn't want to be mean and hateful to my family. I wanted my life back! The doctors told me I would never know what caused me to get Arachnoiditis and CPS, but it was all I could think about. I was becoming overwhelmed by both imagination and reality.

Still, it didn't do me any good to dwell on the negative. Somehow I had to find a way to regain control of my life. I would lose everything and everyone I cared for if I didn't find a way to help myself. Would the insurance people ever get back to me? It was time to hassle them, yet again. This—I could do.

Unlucky enough to have this disease that destroys people, but lucky enough to still be here, I was eventually approved to go to the pain clinic for testing. The doctors would tell me if I could be helped. To my surprise, they really understood about pain. What a huge relief. For the first time since I became ill I wasn't alone with my anguish. Other CPS patients that had the same sort of problems as me, were there being tested. And like me, they were grumpy and hurting. Not that I'd wish this on anyone, but somehow, just knowing others were feeling what I was experiencing gave me comfort.

By the end of the testing, I was told that with hard work, determination and making lifestyle changes I would be able to control my chronic pain, instead of it controlling me. It was a day of tears, but finally, I had some positive news to hold on too. That day a little corner of my very dark world brightened. I now had *HOPE!*

CHAPTER TWO

Finding Help

"The only power we have is the power to change ourselves."
~ Gabrielle Roth

During my search for help I learned that pain treatment centers were opening up all across the country because so many people were being diagnosed with Chronic Pain Syndrome (CPS). I was fortunate to have a pain treatment center close to where I lived. Patients came to the Pikes Peak Pain Program from all over the United States. Many doctors aren't taught how to deal with CPS. It takes a team of medical specialists to help a person whose unrelenting pain has worn down their body and mind. Many days I felt threatened by my own body. At times I was ready to take my own life just to escape the pain.

That first day I visited the pain center, I met with a team of staff members consisting of Dr. John Tyler, the specialist dealing with rehabilitation and chronic pain, Dr. Kevin Murphy, Ph.D., the clinical director, Donna Nyman, counselor and biofeedback therapist, Jane Andrews, the clinical RN, Lisa Molitor, occupational therapist, and Kim Mckeon, the exercise physiologist.

At the end of the testing, these professionals would decide if I was a good candidate for the program. They didn't accept everyone, only the people they knew they could help. I had hit rock bottom, and these were the only people who knew how to help me. Somehow I had to get into this program! My future depended upon it.

It wasn't much fun feeling as if my life was splitting apart at the seams and I couldn't stop it. Dr. Kevin Murphy, Ph.D., the clinical director for the program who did my first interview, put several things into perspective for me. He said the narcotics I was taking were causing me to feel as if I couldn't cope and that this was a normal reaction. I was glad to hear this. At least I knew I was a basket case for a reason someone understood. Though I didn't understand, at least I wasn't losing my mind. I was a victim overloaded by pain and drugs and too consumed reacting to rationalize.

After interviewing with the team of specialists for several hours, I was accepted into the Pikes Peak Pain Program. With proper treatment and hard work on my part, they said they could help me to help myself. In a few months, I would be able to handle the pain and have control of my life again. This seemed unbelievable. At this time the pain controlled everything I thought or did.

I was told that Dr. Higgins and Dr. Tyler from the Pikes Peak Pain Program talked on the phone for more than an hour discussing my diagnosis before I was accepted into the program. Dr. Higgins still looked out for my best interests. I couldn't have a better family physician on my side. Between these two doctors and the rest of the medical team, they decided I had the right attitude. With proper training, I would be a success in the pain management program.

It was liberating to know there was help for a person like me. All this time I had been so alone with my pain. There were others right there at the clinic who had the same kind of problems. I wouldn't wish chronic pain on anyone, but I have to admit I felt better knowing someone else had it too. My world became a little kinder that day, a little less solitary.

Of course, to my dismay, once again, insurance coverage had to be finalized before I could start the program. Nancy Kendrick, M.S.A., CCM, the Case Manager of the clinic would handle the insurance company for me. What a relief! The Case

Manager acts as liaison to insurance carriers, adjusters, attorneys and referring sources. The CM assists in keeping all parties involved informed of progress and recommendations. The CM also provides information and referrals to appropriate community resources. Such resources are designed to support the individual and the family in their efforts to maintain a functional lifestyle in the community.

I wanted to start the next day, but knew that was impossible because of the insurance. It seemed like it had taken forever just to receive approval to come into the pain clinic for testing. I couldn't begin to imagine how long it would take to get permission to actually attend the program. I would just have to wait. Patience is something I've had to learn with chronic pain.

The CM would notify me as soon as she heard from my insurance company. I would have to take more tests to rule out other possibilities. I didn't mind. I had been handed the beginnings of a miracle.

Journal Entry, March 11, 1996

I haven't written for quite some time because everything stays the same as I wait for the corporate structure upon which all medical care is based these days, to put its ducks in a row. I'm still living in pain. Hope is a small thing crouching in a corner of my mind while self-pity and moodiness run wild.

A cleaning lady is coming in once a week because I'm unable to clean my own home. I feel as if my husband doesn't love me, and my children don't need me. Rob says he loves me, that he's only frustrated. I'm frustrated, too. When someone loves you, then you can handle anything life throws at you. At least, that's what I used to think.

I guess I'm being too sensitive. Everything makes me cry. Maybe it's the drugs making me feel so bad. The constant pain is still with me. It amazes me what my body can tolerate. My mind isn't coping nearly as well. Sometimes I think my family would be better off without me. Maybe it's time to pack it in. I wonder if my husband thinks I made myself sick, so I wouldn't have to work. It isn't true. I'm very confused. I'm having a bad mental day.

Waiting for miracles is debilitating.

Journal Entry, March 14, 1996

I had an appointment this morning with Dr. Higgins to discuss my evaluation at the Pikes Peak Pain Management Program. He was happy I had been accepted into the program. These people know about pain. If and when my insurance comes through I can start the program. I'm still waiting to hear if they'll cover me.

Please God! Let this happen!

Today was my youngest son Robbie's birthday and my oldest daughter Aimee's birthday. They were born seven years apart on the same day. Usually I have a big family birthday celebration for my children, but this year I'm not up to it and this makes me feel awful. We had a party, but it wasn't the same.

Some days it's as if my life is already over. Going through this is teaching me to appreciate being able to sit and walk. I have learned to never again take these things for granted.

I have to take more tests. Dr. Higgins and Dr. Tyler ordered blood work and a bone scan. These tests won't be as bad as some I've had to take. Thank goodness!

Finally, after several long weeks of waiting to hear about approved coverage from my insurance company, Nancy, the case manager from the program, called and told me I had been approved. I could start in two weeks. I would be there for six weeks. Each day the clinic would start at 7:30 a.m. and would last until 4:30 p.m., Monday through Friday. If a patient has to miss a day for something less than an emergency, that patient is out of the program. I'm anxious about this rule, but God willing I'll be able to be there every day.

There's a waiting list, and the clinic can only take small groups of patients so everyone can get the individual attention he or she needs. I would have to be serious and dedicated in order for this program to work for me. The good news is I would be able to return home each night to be with my family. This was much better than going into the rehabilitation hospital. I couldn't wait to start. It meant everything to me to actually be able to work with something positive. I'd been in the darkness too long.

Journal Entry, March 18, 1996
Another long pain-filled week and I'm still waiting to start the program. I decided to go by a bar to watch some of my girlfriends who were playing in a women's top ten pool tournament, to determine who is the best female pool shooter in town. The year before, I had placed second in this tournament.

I think it will always bother me to see people doing things I'm unable to do because of chronic pain. I'm forcing myself to try to get out more even though it hurts like crazy. I want to get on with my life. I only stayed a short time because it was too depressing to watch everyone having fun playing pool when I felt so bad.

I needed to get back home so I could lie down and take my pain pills. I hate the way the narcotics make me feel, disoriented and half there. My main goal at the program will be to get off the narcotics as soon as possible. They told me this could happen with hard work and a positive attitude. It's hard to be positive about anything right now. I used to have such optimism. I have to be strong!

Journal Entry, March 22, 1996
My honey surprised me today by taking me to an afternoon movie—such a normal thing for most people, yet for me, it was a special event. Rob knows how much I like to go to the movies, and for a while I could almost believe it was normal for me, too. I enjoyed the movie. We had a good time. I'm lucky to have the love of my life helping me through this ordeal.

It was hard to sit for that long, but I did it. I almost fell down when I got up after the movie, but I didn't say anything. I'm so tired of being in pain, and I know my family is tired of hearing about it.

The pain consumes me. We're all going through changes because of this disease. The pain affects everything I do. It affects my family, friends, and even strangers as well.

The pain interrupts life on every level.

Chronic pain has caused my entire family to go through many changes, some for the good and some not so good. We all have to take it one day at a time. I thank God for my family. I can't imagine going through this alone.

At first, all I did was wonder what caused this incredible pain. Then I denied the fact this had happened to me. I was angry and lashed out at the ones I loved. It didn't seem fair to my loved ones, but that's how chronic pain works.

I would always wonder: Why me?

In most cases, chronic pain is caused by something definitive—some kind of injury, surgery, or a disease. I wondered why it had sneaked up on me without warning or explanation. There were no answers. Mine was not to reason why, but to accept my condition and go on with the healing process.

I couldn't escape the pain, but I could fight it. I refused to let it win. For myself and my family I was determined to get better. I had to believe where there was a will—there would be a chronic pain survivor—*me*.

LINDA'S SUCCESS STORY

Treating Cancer Pain

For about three years, Linda lived with nonstop, severe pain. Diagnosed with multiple myeloma, a form of bone cancer, she suffered from multiple compression fractures of the spine as the cancer progressed. Because of the pain from these fractures, she could hardly walk or get out of bed. Today, Linda's pain no longer slows her down, thanks to Advanced Pain Therapy (APT)Intrathecal.

After being diagnosed with cancer, Linda underwent chemotherapy and radiation treatments to control the cancer and the related pressure on her spine. "Conventional drug therapies, such as pills and skin patches, just didn't provide any pain relief," she said. Nothing seemed to ease her pain.

Then, after just about giving up hope, Linda's oncologist recommended that she visit a pain management specialist who suggested she try APT Intrathecal. APT Intrathecal uses a small pump that is surgically placed under the skin of the abdomen to deliver medication into the intrathecal space, where fluid flows around the spinal cord. The medication is delivered through a small, soft tube that is also surgically placed. The spinal cord is like a highway for pain signals on their way to the brain, where the feeling of pain is experienced by the body. Because APT Intrathecal delivers medication directly to where pain signals travel, pain can often be dramatically controlled with only a small fraction of the dose required with oral medication. This helps minimize side effects.

After a successful screening test, Linda began receiving APT Intrathecal. "I'm so much more comfortable," she said. "I've found a way of controlling the pain that could have ruined the rest of my life." Before receiving APT Intrathecal, Linda was in such pain she rarely left her house. Now she enjoys going out to lunch, visiting with friends, and doing everyday activities that were once impossible because of her pain.

Linda experienced no side effects from the therapy. "This therapy has made a remarkable change in my life," she said. "I'm up and doing things that I haven't been able to do for three years. It's the only treatment that has worked for me."

Will my insurance company pay for Medtronic APT Intrathecal?

The system is approved by Medicare and many insurance carriers will pay for APT Intrathecal. However, as with many therapies, you and your doctor will have to get approval from your insurance company before you can receive APT Intrathecal. Consult your doctor or insurance carrier for more specific information.

CHAPTER THREE

Philosophy of a Chronic Pain Program

"People who have something better to do don't suffer as much."
- Fordyce

Even though there is no cure for Chronic Pain Syndrome (CPS), it can be managed. With proper support and making lifestyle changes patients can come to rely on themselves and live a full rewarding life.

More than 86 million people have been stricken with CPS. And with the Baby Boomer generation getting older, there are many injuries and cases of chronic pain being diagnosed every day. One out of every three people have this condition. I wasn't alone.

Patients are selected for the chronic pain program because they have a certain point of view about their pain and are strong minded. There is a personal responsibility. They have to do things for themselves.

This program assists patients to learn the skills required to manage their problem without depression and anger.

"Medical Model," is a term used to define the medical system. The diagnosis determined why I was having a problem. This could be discovered through various testing such as MRI's, CAT Scans, EEG's, or X-rays. These are all diagnostic tests, however pain is a symptom of my condition, which is called Arachnoiditis. Therefore my treatment was selective.

High tech medical treatment enabled doctors to title my problem. Most people in today's society are impressed with high-tech medical capabilities. I had the attitude that when a physical problem occurred, I could get the treatment through surgery or medication, and I'd be cured. Unfortunately, not this time.

A passive patient is a patient who has no knowledge of what the medical profession is doing to him. In an instant gratification world, surgery or medication is commonly what patients expect, and make no effort to really understand exactly what is happening to them. If a doctor or nurse tells the passive patient to take pills or have this organ removed in surgery, he is usually agreeable to the treatment without question, because he is desperate to find the cure for his ailment. This behavior is ingrained in our society.

But who is responsible for the Medical Model? It is an external point of view created by the experts, but the responsibility of becoming healthy lies with the patients. I was confused and frustrated and didn't know what to ask. There were no guidelines or books on how to reach a cure for my condition. My feelings of fear and anxiety were reasonable feelings, regardless of the effort I displayed.

With intervention, 50% of patients with CPS are able to return to work while without only 2 in 500 can.

I soon learned the chronic pain program was designed to get me in the best possible shape physically and emotionally. It would attempt to help me convert anxiety and fear into energy and motivation. The goal was to help me learn skills to apply to improve my condition. Chronic Pain Syndrome is a disability, and I could learn to function with my disease, not cure it. There is no cure.

I had to forget about the Medical Model attitude I was used to. This attitude consisted of a lack of knowledge. I had to learn to shift my way of thinking to a "Self Help Model." A Self Help Model is based on education about my disease and chronic pain.

Shifting my way of thinking was shifting my personal responsibility. The challenge remained the same for me. I would become more educated about my problem than some of the physicians I would see. This was a way for me to take personal responsibility and learn to shift my thought process. Becoming responsible for myself was a major shift. I could no longer feel victimized.

I was told that when I would leave the Pikes Peak Pain Program I would be off of all narcotics and able to control my pain with exercise, a healthy diet, and a good mental state of mind. I would be on my way to inner peace. I would learn to be a healthier person both physically and mentally. Those words were like a magic healing balm to my wounded soul.

CHAPTER FOUR

Misery Loves Company

"Not to venture is shrewd. And yet by not venturing, it is so dreadfully easy to lose that which it would be difficult to lose in even the most venturesome venture...one's self.

For if I have ventured a miss...very well, then life helps me by its punishments. But if I have not ventured at all...who helps me?" - *Soren Kierkegaard*

With the promise of new hope, the Pikes Peak Pain Program quickly became a major part of my life. I had looked forward to this day for a long time, and now it was finally here—my first day of classes. I admit I was a little nervous and somewhat skeptical.

The philosophy of the program said it all: *"Make the most of yourself, for that is all there is of you."* Being one of my favorite quotes by Emerson, this was a good omen. I was at my wit's end. I had nowhere else to go. This was my last chance to get my life back. The program had to work for me.

Journal Entry, March 27, 1996
I'm in a good mood. Today was the first day of the rest of my new life. I'm in a class with four women and three men. We are all in the same boat. We have Chronic Pain Syndrome.

Today we actually exercised. We started with stretching and walking in the swimming pool. We also lifted one pound weights and worked with some exercise machines in the exercise room at Health South. I'm meeting aching muscles I never knew I had and feel like I've been run over by a truck. God, please give me the strength to stand the pain and help me get through this program.

They are telling us that by learning a new way of living, we can control the pain. They'll be teaching us how to relax. This will reduce the stress, which will reduce the pain.

The others who are in their second week seem to be improving with the program. Everyone seems nice. There is a bond developing between the class members. This is a bond that goes deep, all the way to our soul. We share something no one else can understand. Family and friends are codependents in a sense—victims of our pain. We are fellow warriors, taking back our territory, taking back our lives.

One man in my class was in a body brace and had worn it for several years. He had been crushed in a ditch. He was young, with a wife and two small children. My heart went out to him and what he and his family had been living with for the last three years.

We each have a story to tell. In the end, it's the same result: We all have chronic pain. The others had been there for two to three weeks. The clinic staggered the classes so the veteran students could help the people new to the program. I heard their stories and saw how the program was working for them. To see how they had progressed added to my burgeoning hope.

Hearing strangers talk about their individual situations gave me the courage and strength to open up and share my story. Also, it let me know I was not alone with my pain. The old saying *"misery loves company"* is true. I'm a living, breathing example. When I saw others with bigger problems than I had, it gave me a whole new perspective. If you take the time to look around there is always someone in worse shape than you.

About three hours of mild exercise a day was expected from me. Lectures were spaced around the exercise time, so everything was balanced out. There was no way I could exercise for three straight hours. I didn't know how I would be able to do all this exercise and handle the pain, but everyone else was doing it and this was my last chance. Somehow, I would manage.

'By learning a new way of living I will be able to control the pain,' became my mantra. I repeated it several times a day. I would be learning how to relax through biofeedback. This would reduce the stress, thus reducing the pain. It sounded too good to be true. Controlling the stress was difficult for me. I'd always been the worrier in my family. I had to admit I was skeptical of all this, but I had to succeed in this program. I'd do my best to stay positive about what they were teaching us.

After my first full day, my whole body ached. I still had chronic pain, but also a different kind of pain, a good kind, like I used to feel when I did aerobics or walked a couple of miles. I never dreamed I would be able to exercise again. Of course, this was more stretching and lifting of one-pound weights than the kind of exercise I was used to doing. Before the Arachnoiditis and chronic pain, I used to walk ten miles a week. Now, I was lucky if I could last on the treadmill for five to ten minutes. There were many so things I couldn't do that were easy to do such a short time ago. I had to believe in my heart that God would give me the strength to stand the pain and somehow I would master this program.

The others in my class who were in their second week seemed to be improving. One of the things I noticed about these people was they seemed happy, even with their chronic pain. I asked myself, "How can that be?" When you're being consumed with pain, it's hard to smile. What was their secret? To my amazement, they were actually laughing in some of the classes. This surprised me. How could they laugh when they felt like I did? I couldn't remember the last time I laughed.

I wondered if two weeks could possibly make that much difference for me. The new patients, like myself, were totally exhausted in their pain. At the end of the day, I could see it in their eyes and my own reflection.

Journal Entry, March 30, 1996

The sun is a reminder that every day brings another opportunity. Chronic pain has become a part of my life.

Tonight I am very sore. My whole body is screaming. Or should I say, my muscles are crying out against the exercise and stretches the instructors are teaching me. It's odd, because it can hurt really bad, but feel good, too. It helps to be getting out and doing something positive.

I can't believe how much I actually miss doing exercise. To think I always hated exercise. It feels good to be able to walk on the treadmill, even if it's only for a few minutes. This is about the only thing that feels good. Oh yeah, another thing I like is being in the swimming pool. The warm water makes me feel relaxed.

Today we talked about visualization and techniques of relaxation. It has always been difficult for me to relax. I think now I'm ready to learn how to do this. I have no choice. I have to learn to relax, because when I'm not relaxed I'm stressed. Stress causes muscle tension, which increases pain. I have to learn to control what stresses me out in order to conquer the pain.

Everyone is friendly to me. There is a certain kind of chemistry developing between us. I know it's because of the pain we have in common. It's hard to try to explain to someone who hasn't experienced it. They couldn't possibly relate to this intense pain unless they were feeling it in their own body.

Chronic pain has a way of wearing down my body physically and the drugs dulling my senses making me feel trapped in a useless shell. My mind still works, but it's as if my body has given up. But in the program I see the miracle happening in others. If they can overcome and improve, so can I.

Working hard in my fight, my big accomplishment for the day was learning how to find my neutral spine. This is an area in which I had the least amount of pain, whether lying down, sitting, or standing. Imagine feeling a straight line from the tip of your tailbone to the top of your head. This is your neutral spine, also the proper balanced back posture for yoga. Although I have never practiced yoga, I could feel when my back would slide out of this zone. The exercise physiologist and recreational therapist, Kim McKeon MS, had taught me how to find neutral spine. I hurt terribly, but it felt good to be accomplishing something. I was on my way to getting better.

No matter what the cause of your chronic pain, you too, can find your neutral spine. All it takes is the spark of hope, and the right attitude to get you started....

JOHN'S SUCCESS STORY

Treating Complex Regional Pain Syndrome

"I was so tired of having pain every day. Because I had two grandchildren I wanted to play with I was willing to try the Advanced Pain Therapy (APT) Neurostimulation. Ready to give up, I took a chance, and I won."

John had injured his right shoulder at work while lifting eighty to two-hundred pound slabs of marble. Time off, combined with physical therapy, exercise, and massage he found relief from his pain. But John reinjured his arm when he returned to heavy lifting, and the resulting pain was vicious, extending from his shoulder to his fingertips. "Searing pain, like laying my arm on a hot stove."

John's arm was extremely sensitive to temperature changes and touch. He wore an oversized garden glove on his hand most of the time because he couldn't bear to have anything or anyone touching it. His doctors tried a number of pain medications, antidepressants and anesthetic injections. One year after his injury, John underwent surgery to repair the tear in his shoulder, but the pain remained.

Soon after, he had an APT Neurostimulation screening test, in which a pain specialist placed a lead—a special medical wire at the level of his spine that corresponded to where he felt pain. He experienced 80% pain relief. "I slept all night without taking pain killers for the first time since I injured myself," says John. Two weeks after the screening test, the doctor implanted a permanent neurostimulation system.

Since receiving the system, John says he occasionally experiences some pain, most notably when there is a change in the weather. But this, he can live with. John is now employed full-time and no longer requires any oral medication for pain relief. And he can play with his grandchildren.

What is Medtronic Advanced Pain Therapy Neurostimulation?

APT Neurostimulation, including both spinal cord stimulation and peripheral nerve stimulation, uses a small neurostimulation system that is surgically placed under the skin to send mild electrical impulses to the spinal cord. The electrical impulses are delivered through a lead, a special medical wire that is surgically placed. These electrical impulses block the signal of pain from reaching the brain. Peripheral nerve stimulation works in a similar way, but the lead is placed on the specific nerve that is causing pain rather than near the spinal cord.

Because APT Neurostimulation works in the area where pain signals travel, electrical impulses (which are felt as tingling), can be directed to cover the specific sites where you are feeling pain. APT Neurostimulation can give patients effective pain relief and can reduce or eliminate the need for repeat surgeries and the need for pain medications.

CHAPTER FIVE

Organization - Energy Conservation - Pacing

"Focus all your energy, not on fighting the old, but on building the new." - *Socrates*

If I didn't stand for something, I'd fall for anything. It was time for me to take my stand against Chronic Pain Syndrome.

Pain or injury can use up a great deal of energy. Learning ways to conserve my energy allowed me to put the leftover into activities I enjoyed. And a side benefit was that it also ended up protecting my body. When I was over-fatigued or overdid things, I ended up straining my back or my shoulders. I had to learn a whole new way of performing simple movements that I'd always taken for granted. I had to be conscious of every move so I would do it right and not harm myself.

The basic principles of saving energy are Organization, Pacing, Labor saving devices, and Body mechanics, all which help me conserve my energy. The two most important are Organization and Pacing. Most of us understand the concept of organizing. However, I needed to understand the different aspects of organization.

Organization, when it came to energy conservation, means things like rearranging my kitchen, bedroom, closet or my computer desk to make life easier. I placed things at heights I could reach so I didn't have to strain my back or bend much. I stored things together. A good example; I didn't take my laundry supplies and put all the detergent upstairs away from my washer and dryer, and put my laundry basket in a different room. I kept them by my appliances. I put things together in a systematic order. This saved me time, energy and wear and tear on my body.

The kitchen needed complete reorganization. My pots and pans were stored by the refrigerator and the spices were over by the sink, and I ended up running back and forth to get what I needed. I had to rearrange my house for my own good. That was something I needed to think about. Always looking at things, I would have to ask myself: Is there an easier way to do this?

Pacing and energy conservation meant not giving into my pain. Changing my way of doing things and changing my house boiled down to refusing to let pain control my life. At first, it was very frustrating to think I had to change things for the pain.

No, I'm not going to do that, I'm not going to let this pain get me down. I'm not going to change anything. I'm going to keep on going the way I have been. Thinking like this would only hurt me. I was to the point I hurt so badly I had to accept the pain and change things to help myself. I had to seize every minute of every day to the fullest. That wasn't giving in to the pain. That was learning how to help me deal with it.

I realized then the changes in my home made sense for everybody. When doing things I hated like vacuuming and dusting I played music that was soothing, something that had a nice flow. If I had music playing while I was doing stressful things, like paying bills, I flowed with the rhythm of the music and as a result suffered less stress. This harmony seemed to lessen the pain. It helped the mood and the atmosphere.

Think about ways you can conserve energy. Always sit when possible, unless sitting is a painful position for you. If it's better standing then by all means stand. But sitting is definitely a less energy-consuming position. When I sit down, my body doesn't have to work so hard.

Good lighting also reduces strain. The better my lighting was, the better I could see things. Making it easier on myself, I changed all the light bulbs in my home. Another thing that helped me was making things more accessible. I kept things handy, even in the bathroom. I used to keep mouthwash and hairspray under the sink, where it was hard to reach. I did myself a favor and put up an extra shelf. I put the stuff right where I needed it. It wasn't worth the pain to have to bend for things. Taking action for myself made me feel better.

Journal Entry, April 2, 1996

A pretty good day. I tried to pace myself, but didn't do such a good job. It's going to take practice. Tonight I feel good about increasing my exercise. I don't feel so sluggish. Who would've thought this would happen to me? I have discovered I actually like doing exercise.

I think I would've felt better if I had stopped a little bit sooner. Pacing seems to work. I'm so used to keeping on until I get something finished. It's hard to walk away when there's still something left to do. I have to take breaks and then finish whatever I'm doing later. I have to learn how to stop before the pain comes. That isn't going to be easy. But nothing is worth increasing the pain.

The pain clinic is helping me feel better about myself. They have a lot to offer to people who are in the same physical condition I'm in. Actually, everyone could benefit from what they are teaching us, whether you have pain or not.

In dealing with chronic pain, pacing was the most important part for me to learn. What did I do on good days? I did too much. What did I do on bad days? I did nothing. Pacing did not mean pushing myself on good days. It meant I had to spread my life out between the good and the bad.

Before I went to the pain clinic, good days found me in a great mood. I woke up and even with my pain, I felt good. My family and I started out on a good note. Then they left to go to work and school. I might decide I was going to do laundry or run errands but in the middle of the day my mood turned to crap and when my family came home they would wonder what had happened.

Well, all that happened was that I pushed, pushed, pushed, and caused my pain to increase. I did it to myself. They didn't understand how I could change so fast. And if I wasn't having a good day, then I was having a bad one and took it out on those around me. There was no happy medium. If I paced myself on the good days when I had them, then I'd have more good days in a row. The pain didn't increase, because I wasn't overdoing it. This is what Pacing is all about. Stopping before the pain comes is the most important thing.

Here's an idea to think about. Take a schedule and make a typical day for yourself. Think about your normal routine. Write down what you try to do. Try to plan your day realistically. Just pick a normal day. I had to think about going from a day when I really didn't do anything to a day several months ago when I had a life before chronic pain. I had to pace myself to make it work. In looking back, I realized my normal life before chronic pain was more strenuous than I had thought.

Learning about Pacing led to a more fundamental lesson for me. I realized I had to be kind to myself. If I wasn't good to myself I ended up pushing myself backward instead of forward. When this happened, the family's support was lost. They didn't understand and they paid as high a price as I did.

I had no other choice but to be good to myself. I had to think about me. For awhile, I had to put me first. This is what dealing with chronic pain is all about. I had to make myself happy before I could make those around me happy. That wasn't being selfish. That was taking care of me and my body. Then and only then would I be able to take care of my family. It helped me believe in myself and that belief was wonderful to have.

Pacing is tough for people who tend to overdo it. I tried timing myself. I would work for fifteen minutes at the computer and have to stop because I could feel my pain increasing. When this happened, I had to allow myself time to rest. In the beginning I would have to lie down for about fifteen minutes before I could go back to work. Later, I was able to walk on my treadmill or sit down and have a coffee break.

A few more minutes of work would add to so much pain. I had to take time-outs, or by the end of the day I would be in severe pain. Setting priorities, with my health being top priority, taught me how to pace myself.

I learned I can control the pain with pacing, instead of the pain controlling me. I bought a timer and I broke up the heavy and light work throughout the day. I had to take a few minutes for myself each hour. In the beginning, a general rule was to rest ten minutes every hour. I learned to listen to my body and it told me by way of pain tolerance, when I needed to stop. Walking away from what I was doing made such a difference in the way I felt at the end of my day. I needed to get a short rest, away from people. Finding a quiet place to rest was one of the things that helped me the most. I found I could lighten up on my work and still earn my keep.

I took responsibility in deciding what kind of lifestyle I wanted to live. I had to bring it all together with pacing, energy conservation, and organization. A big realization for me was that my health, pain, or lack there of was up to me. No one else could do it for me. I set my own priorities for my own lifestyle. I prepared myself for my work at home and on the job. I thought about things differently, like how to sit, stand, or walk. I learned how to pace myself and take care of me and my body so I'd have more good days. I learned to pick out things I could do, not things I couldn't do.

With practice I got good at this and so can you!

CHAPTER SIX

Addiction to Prescription Drugs

"Out of the Blue, into the black." *- Neil Young*

I believe we will each have our own season touring through hell. Mine was accepting the fact that I had became addicted to prescription narcotics, and facing the idea that I would have to live with Arachnoiditis and chronic pain for the rest of my life. As Dr. Murphy had told me on that first day, I had to make the most of myself, because that's all I had left.

When I was diagnosed with Arachnoiditis and Chronic Pain Syndrome, I decided I would never succumb to self-pity. To me that was the dreariest of my emotions. Going through my darkest days, sitting in my recliner with the drapes closed, my phone turned off, taking my drugs, I wouldn't let myself give in to the pain, even though I was tempted.

It had been devastating to feel the pain increasing each day and to constantly be losing my abilities to do my normal activities. I was unable to do anything but sit and wonder where it was all going to end. Not knowing where to go for help was the part I feared the most. I was blessed the day my family doctor found the Pikes Peak Pain Program for me.

The difference between acute and chronic pain is that acute pain lasts less than three months and can be cured. Acute pain can be fixed with medication, surgery, or by certain medical treatments.

With surgery, doctors know what kind of drugs to prescribe. The drugs used for acute pain usually include pain medications, such as narcotics. I had the right treatments and medication, yet the pain was still with me. Chronic pain lasts longer than three months, in spite of reasonable treatment. It can't be cured and there is no set drug regimen.

Most doctors aren't familiar with the problems that arise with Chronic Pain Syndrome. Until recently, they haven't been taught very much about chronic pain in medical school. I had taken drugs for six months to a year for acute pain when I actually had Chronic Pain. This was where my addiction grew. Any person who takes narcotics for a year or more becomes addicted. It would take a specialist in the field of chronic pain to know what was best for my condition. I thank God Dr. Higgins helped me get into the pain program. Without help, I would've been lost.

Everything was being prescribed by doctors, so I didn't realize what had happened to me until I had entered the pain program. I thought I was okay. I was caught in the trap of legalized drugs. I soon found out I was addicted to prescription narcotics and I was disgusted.

On my third day at the Pikes Peak Pain program, Dr. Tyler told me that would be the last day for me to be on my medication. From then on, I would be drinking a pain cocktail four times a day, and eventually be weaned off all narcotics. During class the next day, I would be flushing all my medication down the sparkling bowl.

I had to admit I was somewhat concerned about getting rid of all my pain medication. I didn't want to be addicted to the drugs I was taking, yet I had tried on my own to cut back on them but I couldn't do it. It was terrifying to know if the pain increased, I would have no means of relieving it.

I found out later that there would be three of us kicking the drug habit, so I had company in my effort to get off the narcotics. I had heard stories about drug rehabilitation and I was scared. I didn't know if I could stand the pain without the drugs. Just in case I couldn't take it, I was tempted to keep some of my pain pills.

However, I'd made up my mind to succeed in the program and I would do everything they asked of me. I was fearful, but the next day all my drugs went down the drain. Anyway, I hated the drugs. They didn't stop the pain. They only took the edge off and had turned me into a zombie. It had gotten to the point when my children or my husband told me something, five minutes later I couldn't remember it. I was always making some kind of dumb mistake. Dr. Tyler told me that when the time came to get off the pain cocktail, it would be easier than getting off the narcotics. I really wanted to believe him.

On my way home from the clinic I stopped at the pharmacy to pick up my prescription for the pain cocktails. I didn't have any idea what was in them. The next day I took three of the four ounce bottles to the clinic and gave them to Jane Andrews, one of the registered nurses who ran the program. She would give them to me when it was time for me to take them. In the meantime, she kept them locked up in the office.

I thought it must be some powerful stuff to keep locked up. I was so right. Jane gave me my first pain cocktail at seven that morning. Within twenty minutes I felt totally disoriented and sleepy. I could hardly stay awake during the lectures. I need not have been worried about throwing away my medication. Later, I found out the pain cocktails were three times stronger than what I had been taking. This was why I was having such a hard time concentrating in class.

The idea was to wean me off the drugs gradually. Each day the pain cocktails were to become less potent. Eventually, I would be off all medication and controlling my pain through pacing, exercise, biofeedback, managing my stress and many other lifestyle changes I was learning. My major goal in the program was to get off all drugs. And there I was, higher than a kite.

I had my second pain cocktail at 11:00 a.m., and this one made me feel even worse. My stomach felt queasy and I was barely able to maintain my composure. I felt sleepy and disoriented all day. That's when I realized `this was going to be hard. The pain was still there, but I was gone. I had my third pain cocktail at 3:00 p.m. Having a low tolerance for any kind of drug, this was hitting me hard. All I wanted to do was go to sleep, but I couldn't because I had classes until 4:00 p.m. I just wanted to go home. It had been a long day. I hurt all over. I felt lousy.

The last thing I had to do for the day was learn a relaxation technique through Biofeedback. Donna Nyman, the counselor hooked me up to a computer that showed my pain line and a line where it should be when I was less stressed. By breathing correctly and concentrating, I could actually see my pain line come down to a more normal level. That was interesting.

Biofeedback uses electronic feedback to teach patients how to control physical processes, such as reacting to stress by tightening head and face muscles, which may result in tension headaches. Electromyographic biofeedback alerts patients to muscle strain and works especially well for tension headaches and for jaw, neck, and shoulder pain. That day, biofeedback really worked for me.

When I first went into the room, I felt sick to my stomach because of the pain cocktails. The time went by fast and I felt better by the time I left the building to drive home. I actually controlled my level of pain by breathing and concentration.

On the drive home I began stressing. I became caught in heavy traffic and desperately needed to toss my cookies. There wasn't anywhere to pull off the road. I tried to stay calm concentrating on not panicking and keeping my lunch down. The more stressed I became, the worse I felt. Everything I had in me came out all over me, my clothes, and my car. I couldn't stop it; it kept coming. I was misery in its truest form.

Still a few miles from home, it took all I had to just concentrate on driving and arriving home safely. I just wanted to sleep. When I finally pulled into the garage I shook like a leaf in a wind storm. I honked the horn and my daughter Jennifer and my husband Rob came out and helped me out of my car. I was shaky and sick. I could hardly walk. They helped me remove my coat. Luckily, the worst of the mess landed on it. All I wanted was a hot shower and my bed. Jennifer put my things in the washer and helped me to my bedroom. My husband took on the terrible job of cleaning up my car. I knew it was a labor of love on their parts. They were there for me!

After sleeping for a couple of hours, I felt better. I dreaded taking my 9:00 p.m. pain cocktail. I had gotten my stomach settled down and drank some chicken broth and ate some crackers. By that point it had stayed down. I didn't want to go through that again, and I still felt like a space cadet.

I thought this must have been what it was like to be stoned in the sixties and seventies. I grew up in those wild and crazy days. I didn't like drugs then either and I really didn't like the way the pain cocktails made me feel. They were worse than the narcotics I'd been taking. I decided to talk to Dr. Tyler in the morning. I knew I couldn't go on like this.

Rob told me I shouldn't be driving in that condition and I agreed. I had been lucky to have made it home safely. He made the decision to drive me to the clinic each day. So much for my hard earned independence. I took my 9:00 p.m. pain cocktail and fortunately I didn't get sick and actually that night I got a full night's sleep. This was the first time I had slept through the night in about a year. The spasms in my back, hips, and legs would always wake me up. Hummm...maybe the pain cocktails weren't so bad after all.

Dr. Tyler met with each of us every morning before classes to discuss our progress. The next morning when I talked to him he told me I shouldn't be feeling any nausea with the pain cocktails. They called the pharmacy and had them make me up a new batch. I had a low tolerance for drugs and those prescribed had been too strong for me. The new pain cocktails still made me loopy and sleepy, but I could handle these. I'd assumed it would get better as time went by and it did.

Journal Entry, April 3, 1996
One week behind me. I'm beginning to feel better. The pain is still here, but I understand it better. I have actually been able to get a few good nights' sleep. Even though it is drug induced, sleep makes a great deal of difference in the way I feel about things. It's wonderful what sleep does for the body and the mind.

It's amazing how different my outlook is after only one week. Today they told me once again, this pain is forever, it will never go away. I'd been told this before, but it was hard to wrap my mind around. I've been trying to accept this fact for some time now. Dr. Higgins did a good job of preparing me for accepting a life of chronic pain. I owe him a great deal for sending me to the right doctors to get me into this program.

The pain cocktails are still making me a space case, but I'm handling them better. All I can do at this point is take things one day at a time. I am also getting better at controlling my stress. I guess a person can live with just about anything once they're taught how.

They say God never closes the door without opening a window. Sometimes, I think my window is stuck. I have always wanted to do something to help other people. I think I would like to write a book about chronic pain in order to help other people learn how to live with theirs. If it would make it easier for just one person, it would be worth it. Maybe it would help someone else to live their life in a more positive manner.

Star Kemp, a local artist who also had chronic pain, committed suicide this past week. I have to admit I was right there, until I found help in the pain program. There was a long article in the newspaper about him. I wondered if he could have been in this program with the rest of us, maybe that wouldn't have happened.

Chronic pain is something not many people are aware of— especially doctors. They need to know the patient's side of it in order to best treat it. I'll continue keeping my journal and then decide what I'll do at a later date. Right now I have to give all my attention to my health. It would be wonderful if I could help other people with their pain through my experience. In a way it would make what I'm forced to endure worthwhile.

It has been a full week of pain cocktails. They still make me spacey, but I'm grateful for them. Each day they are getting weaker and easier to handle. I feel the pain more, but I've learned by changing my attitude about things and making lifestyle changes that I'm able to control it better. The program is working for me. I feel better mentally and physically than I have in a long time. The pain is still with me, but I'm beginning to understand it. I'll be so happy at the end of the program when I'm off all drugs. I'm sick of taking them.

Learning to live with chronic pain is truly a lifestyle change for me. I wouldn't be able to adapt without a team of professionals to teach me how to do it. I couldn't kick narcotics by myself. I needed professionals to show me the way. They are helping me find the strength to get off the drugs and are teaching me how to live successfully with my pain. I'll never forget the strength and support of the people in my classes and the staff. There will always be a spot in my heart for them.

LARRY'S SUCCESS STORY

Treating Arachnoiditis Pain

At age forty-six, Larry injured his back working while setting up trade show displays. He then developed Arachnoiditis, swelling of the spidery covering that coats the spinal cord. The condition caused severe pain in his back and both legs, numbness in his left thigh, and burning pain in both feet.

He was initially treated with antidepressants, narcotic pain relievers and epidural steroid injections. None of these therapies relieved his pain. Finally he was referred by his neurologist to a pain clinic.

Larry hoped to be able to walk again, increase his activity levels, and decrease his use of pain medication. Since Advanced Pain Therapy Neurostimulation, he has experienced 75% pain relief, is more active and has decreased his oral pain medications. He is now able to sleep at least six hours a night, which has significantly improved his life.

Larry underwent a screening test for Advanced Pain Therapy Neurostimulation, during which a temporary lead, (a special medical wire), was placed at the area of the spine that corresponded with where he felt pain. He experienced seventy-five percent pain relief within twenty-four hours. Because this test was successful, Larry went on to receive a permanent system.

Two years later, Larry continues to experience good pain relief. He has worked with his pain specialist to reprogram the neurostimulation system to cover changes in his pain. Larry is able to walk several blocks with minimal discomfort and is better able to accomplish activities of daily living. Some of his pain remains, but is easily managed with oral pain medications. Larry now sleeps six hours a night, a significant improvement over the two-hour naps in which he had become accustomed.

Will Medtronic Advanced Pain Therapy Neurostimulation completely eliminate my pain?

APT Neurostimulation does not eliminate the source of pain, so the amount of pain reduction varies from person to person. Your screening test will help your doctor see if neurostimulation will work for you. Typically, people who find the therapy helpful experience 50 to 70% pain relief. Those people who do not experience adequate relief generally will not receive a system as part of their pain therapy.

Neurostimulation is just one part in your pain therapy plan. The therapy requires a strong patient commitment to effectively control pain. Learning to operate the neurostimulation equipment and participating in other therapies, such as physical therapy, helps ensure success.

CHAPTER SEVEN

Chronic Pain and How it Affects Others

"There is only one success: to be able to live your life in your own way." *-Unknown*

Chronic pain affected everyone I came in contact with. It affected my family, my friends, and even people I didn't know. When I was wearing a back brace or walking with a cane, most people felt sorry for me. I could see it in their eyes. It was their way of showing compassion to another human being. They would have liked to help me, but didn't know how.

At the Pikes Peak Pain Program they wouldn't let anyone into the program unless they knew the person could do the program—all of it. It was easier for the staff to see my pain and still push me to my limits, because they weren't my family or friends. The patients were screened; injuries, ailments and previous tests were reviewed, and then they were retested before they entered the program, so no one would get hurt by participating. Depending on their injury or situation, each person had their own individual set of exercises and requirements laid out for them.

The clinic took a firm stand about participating in the program. Even if I was reporting increased pain, which most new patients do, that wasn't a reason for not doing what was required of me. This was why it's called Pikes Peak *PAIN* Program. The staff knew I hurt and they wanted to help me make it better, but to do so meant setting new limits and working muscles that hadn't been worked for a long time. I knew it would get worse before it got better. Improvement would come with a high price of hard work and perseverance.

When your loved ones are hurting, it's hard to understand what they are going through. My family didn't know how to help me because they'd never been trained in this area. A lot of times they could see how much pain I was in, but didn't know what it felt like.

They almost wished they could experience what I was feeling, so they would know where I was coming from. It was difficult for them to know what to do or to know whether or not they should be more helpful.

Sometimes families tend to do too much out of love. The more helpful the family becomes, the more helpless the person with chronic pain becomes. In the beginning, it's easy to become caught up in this pattern, which is more harmful than good.

One of the downsides: it focuses everything on the pain and suffering and doesn't allow the person to do the things they can do. This is a reasonable, caring response from families. When people have acute pain, which is different from chronic pain, they are helped by having someone prepare meals for them, take out the trash, clean their house, or by doing whatever they need.

They are relieved of their responsibilities. When I was in my house and doing nothing, I didn't feel good about myself. The things I could do made me feel better about myself. When I wasn't allowed to do the things I could do, I became depressed.

With chronic pain, it's a whole other ball game. Often it's difficult to get people to do the things they can do because they're afraid of increasing their pain. When I started with the pain program I really didn't want to do a lot of things they asked me to do for that very reason. I didn't know what I was getting into. I found out the schedule was tight and it was more work than I had bargained for, but it was my last chance and somehow I had to persevere.

Over a short period of time, I saw the point of the program. I learned a lot and accepted their philosophy, because it helped me to make a lifestyle change, which isn't an easy thing to do. Family members don't have the leverage the program does. I accepted the program. I wanted to be there because I was open-minded and I wanted help and this was the place to get it.

The staff working within the pain program were focused on personal responsibility. They taught me that chronic pain is each individual's problem. The solution to that problem lies with the individual and not with anyone else. They were right. They couldn't help me with my chronic pain unless I decided I wanted to buckle down and learn what they needed me to learn.

It was hard for my family to understand, because they knew habits were hard to break. They knew the habits I had gotten into with my pain were not good for me, like sitting in my recliner and letting life pass me by. However, experts say it takes only six weeks to develop a new habit. I knew it wouldn't be easy to change, but I could do it. Sometimes, when my family could see me come home suffering and in pain from my day at the clinic they thought the staff at the pain program was too tough on me. It was almost unbearable for them. At first they didn't know what was going on.

Journal Entry, April 7, 1996
I had a pretty rough day. It was my misunderstanding; I thought I would be pain free in seven months to a year. But the program couldn't eradicate my pain. They could only teach me how to control the pain. I would never be pain free. It's hard to really accept this fact. I thought I had worked this out in my mind, but I guess the drugs keep me pretty mixed up.

They changed the pain cocktail, and now I'm having an allergic reaction to it. I have developed an itchy rash which acts up when I get into the swimming pool. It doesn't hurt, but I look like I have measles. Ha! Ha! At least I've found my sense of humor. I can laugh at it. A rash is nothing compared to what my body is going through.

I get deeply depressed. Today was hard. It was family day, and I had no one there. They said my family needed to be there. I'll get through it somehow. The kids are in school and Rob has to work. We have so much up in the air with me not being able to work. All this financial stuff makes things harder to deal with, as if I need any more stress in my life. Enough of this boo-hoo stuff. I need to just let it go. It will all work out.

Journal Entry, April 21, 1996

It was snowing outside when I went to the clinic this morning. In spite of knowing how difficult it would be for my family to show up for family day, I kept going to the door to watch for them. I really needed them there. I needed them to see what I was doing and to understand why. I hoped that it would help them understand when I need time alone or when I'm having a bad day. Since my participating in the program adds more strain on them, I guess I need the validation of their approval for the program. I can't deny their attendance would also be an assurance they took all this seriously.

Pain breeds insecurities and doubt. I wonder how anyone can love me when I am so much less than I was before chronic pain? Irrational, I know, but pain is irrational. So are people— for instance the friends who were afraid to be near me for fear that it might somehow rub off on them. Or the friends who had simply gone on without me as if I were expendable. It's terrible to feel so insignificant.

I believe in my heart my family will come.

When my family walked into the room, it made my day. Then I was told they had been there for a while. They'd been in the gym shooting baskets because I was in class. More than anything they could have said, their presence convinced me my doubts were unfounded.

We're going to be all right. It's going to take time and hard work on all our parts. Talking about chronic pain and hearing the other families talk about how it's affecting their lives has opened my family's eyes to what's happening to me. Knowing they weren't alone in having to cope and adjust to living with someone with chronic pain helped them as it had helped me. It hadn't really occurred to me until then that they might have felt just as badly as I had felt, before joining the program.

Rob and the kids said they won't miss any more family days; that it helped them to understand what I was doing and they wanted to be there for me. I was relieved and lucky to have such a family. There was one man going through the program alone and we patients were all there for him. He did just fine without family, but it had to be hard. I thank God for my family. When it comes right down to it, nothing matters but your loved ones.

Each Friday the families came into the clinic for a potluck lunch to become acquainted with the other participants, their families, and the staff. It was important for my family to come on family day to see where I was spending my time and what my different activities were each day I was away from home. It was an invaluable experience for them to see others caught in the same situation and feeling the same frustrations.

We would have open discussions where things were brought up by other families, as well as my own, that needed to be exposed to the light. Sometimes these were things that were hard to talk about with my loved ones. I began to understand their side of it. Mom couldn't do housework, cook, or care for them. They had to step up and it was more work and hard for them too. I'm ashamed to say that until that moment, I saw their problems only as they affected me, rather than how they affected my entire family. After all, they weren't in pain. They weren't incurable. They could live as they wished without impediment. Simple functions that were difficult for me were natural and easy for them. They performed them almost unconsciously.

I realized pain and illness insulates the patient, and it is a natural inclination to allow it. I was so focused on my body, my pain, my responsibility to deal with it, that I failed to see beyond it. I'd become self-centered to survive. I was going to have to expand my focus as it related to my pain to include the viewpoints and problems of my family if I wanted to move beyond surviving and begin to live again.

The effect of chronic pain on families takes its toll. They need to be taught how to live with their loved one who has chronic pain as much as the person living with the pain needs to broaden their focus to include their family. They need to learn how to accept and understand what could help or harm their loved one.

Most people think chronic pain is something that can be fixed. We've all been taught medical science can fix whatever is wrong with us. All the people in the pain program were people that medical science couldn't fix because there is no fix. It's sad, but most families and patients, (me included), take a long time to *really* accept their situation.

From here on out, I had a different point of view. I had been used to a passive role where I went to the doctor and the expert did something to me. Nine times out of ten, I didn't understand what they were doing because they used big words, but since they made me feel better, I didn't bother to ask. It was a mystery to me why I was better, but being better was all I cared about.

People who live with chronic pain with no help tend to isolate themselves from the world around them, including their family. That was my case in the beginning. I wanted to be left alone with my pain. My family had adapted, but it wasn't good for them or me.

Racked with pain, I went into my own little world. I was grumpy and had forgotten how to laugh. I wanted only to stay in my bedroom alone. This wasn't a good avenue for my personal relationships. Sometimes the distance was so great it turned into real trouble and I felt lost to my family and friends. I was lucky they stood by me.

One of the advantages of having so many people in the pain program with the same problem was that I couldn't escape the truth. I learned to accept the fact I had chronic pain and it was up to me to decide how I wanted to live with it. I knew it would never go away.

It was very hard to let go of the idea I couldn't be fixed. I'd always been told they had something that would really help me, whether it was surgery, drugs, acupuncture, acupressure, or a chiropractor.

Most patients had been told, "I know what's wrong with you, just come into my office and we'll fix you. Then you'll be as good as new." I wanted to believe this because I was so tired of the pain.

In most cases, families get their hopes up just to be disappointed. It's vital the family accept the fact that chronic pain is forever.

One thing that helped to control the pain was teaching my family not to focus on my pain. I asked them not to mention the P word. They didn't ask how my pain was or how my back felt on any given day. I had to educate my family not to draw attention to my pain.

My family made some rules. I talked about how my day went, pain wise, then I dropped it. It was hard when I was in pain, and looked like I was in pain, to dissuade the family from running to get me a pillow or doing other things that drew attention to the problem. It took time to educate them to the way I wanted them to react. I had to be patient with them.

My behavior as a person in pain became so subtle, usually only a family member would pick up on it. Of course, their first instinct was to try to make it better for me.

Another person couldn't ask how my back was without getting back to the thing which I was trying to get away from. It was like a Catch-22. For my friends, it seemed like such an understanding, caring thing to do. However, it still focused on the problem.

It was hard to stop talking about my pain because it had become my way of life. I was trapped in this anguished body with nowhere to go. Talking about it had become a habit. One I had to learn to break. And that took time and self-discipline. Even when approached by co-workers, friends, or strangers, I felt obligated to explain. The questions asked by other people who were unaware of my pain was "How are you doing today?" I had to answer either with the truth or a lie. Either way, it drew more attention to my pain.

Some explanations were functional, such as in the cases of talking to my doctors or therapist. It was all right to talk about it to them. Other times, explanations were non-functional. I had to ask myself if this person would be having this conversation with me if otherwise.

People are more inclined to draw attention to people who are doing badly, and aren't interested in people who are doing great. I had to develop skills to answer these questions about my condition. I sometimes had to say, "I don't wish to talk about it." This was a difficult thing to do, but if I was easy on people, I wouldn't progress. I needed to educate not only my family, but the people around me on how to react to my condition. As long as I did it in a kind way, they understood.

These were examples of things I could take control over simply by saying that I didn't wish to talk about it. There were some things I couldn't control and those caused me to worry, which was non-productive and only caused me more pain. Instead I needed to exercise problem-solving techniques with issues over which I had control.

Caring is a behavior that affected my thought process. It was different from worrying. I cared about my children getting ill, but worrying about this was non-productive. I could react to their situation after it happened, instead of worrying before it happened. I had to make a conscious choice not to worry about uncontrollable situations. I had to learn to let go of harmful thought processes. Worrying about issues wouldn't prevent negative situations from happening.

Problem solving allowed me to think about my options. Taking measures to eliminate unnecessary worry could be as easy as removing dangerous obstacles from a child's reach so it didn't harm itself.

Developing skills to control my thought process drew less attention to my pain, and became a preventative measure. I had to remember chronic pain affected not only myself. This ailment affected my family and friends—even complete strangers. By using what I had learned, my life started getting better.

CHAPTER EIGHT

Strategies of Managing Stress

"I'm certain of nothing, but the holiness of the heart's affections and the truth of the imagination." *-John Keats*

Thinking is critical. Thinking is causality. Thinking causes feeling and feeling causes behavior, good or bad. Being upset or angry caused me more stress, which caused me to have muscle tension, which in turn resulted in pain. By learning to control my anger, I could control the stress, which helped to control the pain. Only *I* could take charge of the way I felt and control the pain in my life. This was my personal responsibility.

I use the term "strategies of managing stress" because it is a conscious thing. As in billiards, chess, or checkers, I had to think it out before I could make my first move. Commercials suggest ways of handling stress such as eating, smoking, drinking, shopping, and taking over-the-counter drugs.

Most of these ways are escape strategies; to obliterate or get away from stress, to cover it up. Every once in a while is fine. However, if I escaped on a regular basis, it would be harmful to me.

Relief was just a swallow away. I wanted peace. I wanted to get out of my pain-wracked body. I wanted to stop the turmoil. I wanted to stop the pain. With the dynamic approach to handling stress, I had great potential to change my life if I chose to take the responsibility. I had always made choices, now this one was up to me. It was time to take responsibility for my pain and I had to stop feeling sorry for myself and get on with it.

There are many ways and strategies of managing stress. Some people do it very well. Some people do it so-so. It wasn't as if I'd never done this before.

Some ways to manage stress are:

- Close your eyes and try to get focused or centered
- Exercise
- Breathe deeply
- listen to music
- Meditate

I like to get close to nature and go up in the mountains. I live in a beautiful part of the country; in Colorado Springs, Colorado. Sometimes I cry, and that's okay. Sometimes I have to let it out and crying is a form of venting, rather like a dryer outlet.

There was so much psychology wrapped up in how I dealt with my pain and I sought answers there as well. For example, Sigmund Freud thought an individual with a closed energy system would mean someone with a troubled childhood, a troubled home, complexes, and defenses.

I had heard about this stuff in college in Psychology 101. When someone said I was being defensive, it was a psychoanalytic term. I even knew some of those defenses were denial, rationalization, and rejection. I didn't know much about psychology, but I knew what those words meant. They had tremendous influence because of the suggestion I had to get all this stuff out of my system. People have been told they would have to lie down on a couch and sort a lot of this stuff out two times a week for two or three years, and then and only then, can they lead a reasonably authentic life. Freud was a very pessimistic fellow. He thought the best a man or woman could do was to get all this crap out and muddle through life.

A lot of psychologists and psychiatrists didn't agree with Freud, but he had tremendous influence. So when I talk about venting that's where the term comes from, as if I were a pressure cooker. It's a very simple principle. I would build up pressure inside a pot and it cooked everything faster. When it built up too much pressure, I had to let some off steam through the smokestack on top. I had to vent it.

That's the way Freud viewed emotions, stress, anger, and internal conflict. His solution was to blow off this stuff. In the pressure cooker analogy, he focused on the little vent on top. He thought most people's vents were plugged. So in order to get well, I would have to get unplugged. This is over simplification, but I think it's pretty accurate. This stuff would come out like rotten psychological puss. Once it was all out, I'd feel a whole lot better.

Freud wasn't very behavioral; he didn't acknowledge people's lives were still trapped after going through all this stuff. He was mostly interested in the process he called "working through."   He didn't rate it by levels of improvement. I think he got lost in the "working through" process himself.

So when I thought of managing my stress by crying or screaming at the top of my lungs and called that venting, it was quite typical, but I didn't think it was enough. I could imagine a pressure cooker with a huge flame under it and when I spent all my time trying to vent it, I was doing nothing but releasing steam. The simple solution would've been to turn the flame down. Freud didn't have the mechanism to turn the flame down, because he thought the brain was fixed from childhood. I didn't believe that. I believed whoever I was today obviously had a lot to do with how I was raised, but also by what I'd learned and achieved. I am a self-made woman. I can change! I can change beyond recognition if I want to put in the effort.

A lot of strategies for stress are based on venting. Let's say, I had a busy day today. I had things to do, so I wasn't going to go for a drive or to the top of a mountain. I wasn't going to scream at the top of my lungs for fear my next door neighbor would hear my screams and call the police.

I could cry, but if I spent a lot of time crying it would get in the way. I had things to do and places to go and schedules to meet. So I really didn't have the opportunity for venting. I didn't have the time or strength to run six or seven miles a day, or do aerobic exercise at target heart rate. Taking twenty minutes at least three times a week, would've taken too much time. Not many people have time to vent this way, and with my pain it was out of the question.

Anyway, some of the strategies were great and I happened to utilize them. One of the things that helped me was to go for walks by myself. It really helped me, but it was a limited utility. Every time I became anxious, I couldn't just pick up and leave to go for a walk. If I did, nobody would ever see me. Because of my responsibilities, I couldn't always get away.

I had used my pain medication as a way of escaping from reality, but had not labeled the behavior as a strategy. I knew the medication took the edge off, it worked for a while. It gave me the illusion of feeling better.

When I got a feeling of anxiety, I had to do something about it. That was the point. I was never going to have zero anxiety, that's impossible.

I learned about stress and relaxation. I talked to my friends and asked them how they handled stress. It amazed me. Interviews were an interesting exercise for me, if nothing else. Some people used drugs or alcohol or TV. A lot of people watched TV to unwind. It works for some people and not for others. The commercials suggested ways to handle stress such as eat, smoke, drink, shop, and take over-the-counter drugs.

I looked at these ways of managing stress. They are mostly external behaviors perceived as stress reducers. In fact, these are escape strategies. They might work short term, but not for the long haul.

Drinking is a big escape strategy. I don't have anything against alcohol, but it isn't an anti-stress strategy. It wouldn't work for me, because I was on heavy medication and it's not a good thing to combine drugs and alcohol. Booze might have helped for the short time, but would've only made things worse in the long run. Drinking is a deeply ingrained strategy, highly encouraged in this society.

Any Friday, I could go to any bar, in any city, almost anywhere in the world and find people who go to Happy Hour. Why were they at Happy Hour? They'll usually say they've had a hell of a week and are there to unwind, which meant managing their stress.

I liked to go to Happy Hour. Sometimes we would go as a group from work and we had a great time. But if this had been the only way to manage my stress, I would've been in big trouble.

A lot of people in the United States are in debt. They cover up their stress by buying things. This escape strategy can get totally out of hand.

If I wanted to manage my stress better, I had to take my personal responsibility and my actions needed to be improved. I couldn't rely on others and have success. I had to allow myself time to try different methods and give myself time to discover what worked for me.

I wasn't into denial. Denial meant suppressing my feelings. In the beginning, I admit I'd reached the denial state. I fooled myself into pretending to other people what was really going on. The strange thing was that I believed what I was pretending. I was only fooling myself.

With the dynamic approach to handling my stress, I had great potential to change my life. That is, if I chose to take responsibility. If not I would be in danger of the pain wining. I wasn't concerned much about things I had no control over, things that might have happened when I was four or five, the traumatic stuff.

However, I believed the things that happened yesterday, and today, and right now are the things that are really important. I had to consider whether I thought I could change. This is extremely important.

I have a tendency to be high strung to begin with. That is one reason why I have chronic pain. I tend to push, push, push, beyond my abilities, and eventually my zeal catches up with me in the form of Arachnoiditis and chronic pain. I think if I would have stopped there, saying that's just the way I am, I've always been this way, you can't teach an old dog new tricks, I would have been lost.

Some people would've said, "That's just the way I am and I'm proud of it. I don't want you messing around with my head. I don't believe in this psychological stuff." To tell you the truth, there were some things I didn't believe in either.

The question I was getting to was, how was I doing? Was I fine? If I was anxious—and I knew what anxious was like—especially over time, it would wear down my body. I wanted relief from that.

As long as I looked outside myself, I wouldn't solve my problem. The anxiety stemmed from within me. I was a manufacturer of my own anxiety. Like the pressure cooker, I was the one who regulated the heat. I regulate it right here, inside my body, with my thinking. If I wanted to have a lot of heat I was going to feel pretty rotten. If I could discover how to turn this down a little bit I would feel amazingly free and in more control.

In my life, bad things can still happen. Once I realized things were beyond my control, like my children or my husband, who I love dearly, it helped me understand anxiety better. I don't have any control of what happens to them. I do all I can to keep them safe, but things will happen, like getting a terrible disease or getting hit by a car. I can't do anything about that. The events in one's life just come in waves in some random pattern. I had to realize what I could control and let go of the rest.

Journal Entry, April 13, 1996
I don't feel like writing today. I have too much to think about. Rob and I got into an argument about money. It hurt me when he told me to get a job when he knew I couldn't work. I feel so useless. God, what am I going to do? My life is ruined.

Journal Entry, April 14, 1996
My attitude is better today. I thought about things and I know he didn't mean what he said yesterday. I'm proud of myself for not letting the stress of that emotion raise my pain level. I'm getting better at not dwelling on things which cause my pain to increase. Only a short time ago that would've hurt so bad, and I would've dwelled on it for days. This time I was able to let it go in a couple of hours. I won't let anyone hurt me again.

A strange thing happened this morning. Some young woman called and said, "Three gang members broke into my husband's 66 Mustang while parked in front of our office and stole his wallet out of the glove compartment. All his credit cards and the Mustang registration was in it." I was stunned, probably in shock, but I took it well.

This girl said she knew of us because of our property management business in the area and that these guys had also stolen her mom's credit cards. The guys wanted to buy new rims for their car, but the dealer wouldn't take our credit card. She had stolen her mom's and Rob's credit cards back from them. She said if I would bring her a reward, she would give me my husband's wallet back with all the papers in it. The guys had taken the cash.

I thought about calling the police, but decided against it. Surely, I could handle an exchange with a kid at McDonalds. I didn't want to risk not getting Rob's wallet back. There were several irreplaceable pictures of our children in it. It was a scary experience because I couldn't get in touch with my husband. He had gone out of town on business with an associate and was out of cell phone range.

Rob had left the windows rolled down in the parked car outside our office. The mustang was still where he had parked it that morning. Apparently, the young men had taken the things out of the glove compartment and did no other damage.

I knew this girl had his wallet, because he did keep it in the glove compartment of the car. I went to McDonalds and got his driver's license, credit cards and everything back for a small reward.

I was nervous about the exchange on the way to McDonalds. My pain level did escalate. All in all, I handled it better than I ever would have before. I was learning courage from living with chronic pain.

When I returned home, I listened to a relaxing classical tape and slowed down my breathing. It made me feel a lot more relaxed. This experience taught me the breathing techniques really did work. There was hope for me yet.

Today, at the clinic, they told me the reason why I crave sweets was because of the withdrawal from the drugs. Another thing I was surprised about, my headaches were caused because of withdrawal from caffeine. I had been told caffeine *increased pain, so I was staying away from it. The side effect will be a headache until it is entirely out of my system.*

As I learned to manage my stress better, I became committed to having less stressful events in my life so that I'd be much more efficient, could drive better, plan better, and use better judgment. By doing this, my body would be in better shape. I didn't want to end up with my body shot by the time I was fifty-five, and this was where I was headed. I heard this had happened to a lot of people. They got emphysema, ulcers, high blood pressure, or cardiac problems when they were fifty-five or sixty, and their body was done for. I only have one body so I have to take better care of myself while I can.

I have lots of reasons to manage my stress better. Ironically, one of them is to try to manage the events in my life. For instance, when someone cut me off on the freeway, I had to learn to let it go. If I kept thinking about it and dwelling on it, I was only hurting myself. If I really got upset, I could have caused an accident or killed myself or someone else. Most likely, the person who cut me off was already home enjoying their dinner. Whereas I had been internalizing it and hurting myself.

I was learning how to let things go. Managing stress was working for me. It isn't easy to turn the other way when some idiot is calling me names and giving me a hard time on the road. However, for my health and my family, I found it in my best interest to ignore the person rather than give him control over me and my reactions. He was an accident looking for a place to happen. I didn't have to give him the opportunity to include me.

I had to remember; anger equaled stress, which equaled muscle tension, which equaled PAIN! I could control how I felt and thought about what happened. It is the thinking and dwelling on an event that causes pain, so I had to learn to let go of it so I could feel better. It was up to me to take the responsibility to control my anger and stress.

We make choices in life; this one was up to me. It was the time to take responsibility for my own pain. In yet another way, I had to stop feeling sorry for myself and get on with my life.

All journeys begin with one step. I had to see how many more I would take before I would trip. I had to expect this to happen. When I'd fall, I'd pick myself up and start over. I'd take what I learned and make of it all I could. Healing is a solitary matter which must be taken seriously.

RITA'S SUCCESS STORY

Treating Abdominal Pain

"Nobody should have to go through what I did," said Rita. "Pain encompassed my whole life."

Although she never would have chosen the role, thirty-seven year old Rita—a nurse and mother of three children—became a firsthand expert on pain. Her experience began on a snowy hill one day when she was sixteen years old. Her toboggan collided with a tree, resulting in a ruptured spleen and emergency surgery. The operation to remove Rita's damaged spleen proved to be just the beginning of a long cycle of chronic, debilitating pain.

Due to scar tissue—adhesions that form in the body after surgery—Rita suffered bouts of severe abdominal pain for fifteen years. She underwent more than ten surgeries and other treatments to relieve the pain, including oral medications and nerve blocks. Most treatments worked temporarily, but her intense pain always returned.

Rita consulted with various physicians, some of whom told her the pain from the scar tissue was imaginary. She felt hopeless, and considered suicide.

"All I could think about was getting through the pain," Rita said. "It was very rough on the whole family."

Finally, a physician specializing in pain management told Rita about Medtronic Advanced Pain Therapy Intrathecal. One month after a successful screening test, Rita underwent surgery to begin APT Intrathecal. She experienced no complications, and went home the day following the procedure.

"Today my life is a total turnaround," Rita reports. "My pain is gone, and I'm doing what I love to do. I take care of my house and three children. I coach two soccer teams, and I love being able to go out and have fun again. I've ridden roller coasters, and I've even been back on a sled."

Rita occasionally experiences a minor, dull ache in her abdomen, which she takes care of with naxpropen sodium tablets, Aleve, available without a prescription. She has experienced no side effects from the therapy.

Rita hopes to return to work, using her nursing background to help other patients with pain. Her plans include starting a pain support group with the help of her doctor.

"My fourth-grader said to me, 'Ma, you're doing everything you want. You're not lying in bed anymore,' Rita said. "He's right. My child isn't taking care of me. I take care of things myself. I'm living life on my terms."

What happens if the pump runs out of medication?

If the pump runs out of medication, your pain will return and you may experience withdrawal symptoms. Your doctor or nurse can tell when the pump will run out of medication by checking the pump with the programmer during your regular refill appointment and will schedule a refill appointment for you before that time. Make sure you write the date on your calendar and keep the scheduled appointment. In the event that you forget the date, the pump has an alarm to let you know when it is running out of medication. It emits a soft, high-pitched beeping sound repeated several times per minute. It is important to have your pump refilled before the alarm sounds. If you hear the alarm sound, call your doctor for an immediate refill appointment. Some people are unable to hear the alarm, so it is important to notify your doctor if you notice a change in pain relief or other changes.

CHAPTER NINE

Exercise and the Rules of Being Human

"The great art of life is sensation, to feel that we exist, even in pain." *- Lord Byron*

Carefully controlled activity is frequently the right prescription for people with chronic pain. There's no cure for the condition, but a lot can be done to manage it. An exercise program would be necessary for me to maintain what the Pikes Peak Pain Program was teaching me. When I leave the program I will have my own individual exercise program worked out for me. I can join a Health Club or set up an area at home to continue with this all important job of keeping my body as healthy as possible.

It depends on my own personal feelings about where I want to do my exercises. I have been taught an exercise program I must continue for the rest of my life when I leave the clinic. I will never be able to stop doing what I've learned, but that isn't a problem as the exercise makes me feel better.

Journal Entry, April 6, 1996
I'm very sore today. I really feel bad. I hurt more than usual. The classes were good, but I feel awfully grumpy for some reason. I have a crick in my neck and it hurts. As if I

*needed any more pain. Whine, whine, whine, I'm having a
lousy day. I'll keep it to myself. I have to look for something
positive. I've worked my time on the treadmill up to fifteen
minutes for a half mile. This makes me feel better. It will get
better with time. I think I want to get the weights and a tread
mill to use at home.*

*It looks like I'll be here for another three weeks. I'm going
to handle this and learn to control the pain. I refuse to let it
control me anymore. When I think there's no way I can go on,
then another day goes by, then a week, and I'm still here and
looking back. Things are getting better. I just have to stay
focused.*

When I entered the pain program, I wasn't in good physical
condition. My body was deteriorating right before my eyes. I
could barely walk without my cane or assistance. Due to the
pain, I had to stop doing any type of exercise. Before I was
diagnosed with Arachnoiditis and chronic pain, I used to do
aerobics three times a week and walk ten miles. I didn't
appreciate what I could do, as far as exercise, until it got to the
point where I couldn't do it anymore. When I entered the
program I thought I would never be able to exercise again. I
wasn't able to work and I couldn't do many of the household
chores that I used to do so easily.

The pain program helped me set realistic goals for myself.
The main goals of the exercise program were to:

*Increase my activity level and endurance

*Decrease my limitations

*Help me return to my former activities and
interests

*Help me feel better about myself

They taught me to achieve these goals through a variety of
approaches   that   included   stretching,   strengthening,
cardiovascular, conditioning, low-impact aerobics, increased
body awareness, posture and body mechanics, and as
appropriate, decrease gait deviations, and unnecessary
dependence on ambulatory aids. I was able to discard my cane
and back brace in the first week.

The role of exercise in the treatment of chronic pain is a lifelong commitment, but that's okay. When I exercise, endorphins are released by nerves in my brain. Endorphins are the body's natural pain killer. They have the same powerful effect as a drug such as morphine. Individuals produce different amounts of endorphins and this can possibly explain why people tolerate pain differently. The bottom line is that exercise makes me feel better.

I needed a professional to help me set up my individual exercise program. Each person is different and depending on the ailment, one may be able to do exercises another cannot. It was imperative I got on the correct program so I wouldn't cause more damage to my body. I had to remember once I started my program it was a lifelong commitment. Actually, it made me start feeling good about myself and I didn't want to quit so that wasn't a problem. I started to look forward to my exercise program because it made me feel good.

When a person with chronic pain considers an exercise program they should not attempt to do so until they have a program laid out for them by a qualified Exercise Physiologist. I can't stress how important it is to get your own program designed especially for you. GET YOUR DOCTOR'S APPROVAL BEFORE TRYING ANY EXERCISES!

During my time at the pain program, we were given a handout sheet containing the rules on being human. I don't know who the author is, however I would like to share it with those of you who are dealing with chronic pain, whether you are experiencing illness or caring for a loved one who is ill. If nothing else, it will give you something other than pain to think about.

THE RULES OF BEING HUMAN

1. YOU WILL RECEIVE A BODY.
You may like it or hate it, but it will be yours for the entire period of this time around.

2.*YOU WILL LEARN LESSONS*.

You are enrolled in a full-time informal school called *LIFE*. Each day in this school you will have the opportunity to learn lessons. You may like the lessons, or think them irrelevant and stupid.

3.*THERE ARE NO MISTAKES, ONLY LESSONS*.

Growth is a process of trial and error: Experimentation. The "failed" experiments are as much a part of the process as the experiment that ultimately "works."

4.*A LESSON IS REPEATED UNTIL LEARNED*.

A lesson will be presented to you in various forms until you have learned it. When you have learned it, you can then go on to the next lesson.

5.*LEARNING LESSONS DOES NOT END.*

There is no part of life that does not contain its lessons. If you are alive, there are lessons to be learned.

6.*"THERE" IS NO BETTER THAN "HERE*."

When you're "there" has become a "here", you will simply obtain another "there" that will again look better than "here."

7.*OTHERS ARE MERELY MIRRORS OF YOU*.

You cannot love or hate something about another person unless it reflects something you love or hate about yourself.

8.*WHAT YOU MAKE OF YOUR LIFE IS UP TO YOU.*

You have all the tools and resources you need. What you do with them is up to you. The choice is yours.

9.*YOUR ANSWERS LIE INSIDE YOU.*

The answers to life's questions lie inside you. All you need to do is look, listen, and trust.

10. *YOU WILL FORGET ALL THIS.*

11. *YOU CAN REMEMBER IT WHENEVER YOU WANT*.
—*Author Unknown*

CHAPTER TEN

Pain Behavior

"If you don't know the kind of person I am and I don't know the kind of person you are a pattern that others made may prevail in the world and following the wrong god home we may miss our star." — *William Stafford*

Pain behavior is any behavior that indicated to another person I had pain. One of the hardest things for me to do was to ask for help when I was in pain. If I didn't ask, then I wasn't being true to myself and I couldn't grow. On the downside, if I didn't ask for help, then I started feeling sorry for myself, and it was awfully hard to dig out of that hole. The fact that I wanted to be healed right then and there wasn't going to happen. A fact that was very difficult to accept.

Sometimes I'd fall back into the anger or denial phase and want to choke someone, but there wasn't anyone to choke. All I had was myself. I didn't want to take it out on my family. They wanted to help me, but didn't know how when I behaved like that.

I couldn't change yesterday, but I could change today, one minute at a time. It was hard to discipline myself not to show the pain, but it could be done. Character is defined as who I am when nobody is looking. I kept developing character.

I had no choice, but to learn a different way of life. I had to ask for what I needed. I might not get it, but if I asked for what

I needed I was being true to myself. This gave me a feeling I was not a weak person. I needed this support until I could become healthy again.

Everyone with chronic pain needs support from family and friends. It was hard to rely on them when I was experiencing so much pain and although I wasn't generally a burden to them, I sometimes felt like one.

"I'm of no use to anybody, not even myself. What am I going to do with the rest of my life?" Those were some of my negative thoughts. I had to stop those when they came into my mind. I had to remind myself there is a positive side to everything negative. I had to dig deep and look for it.

One part of my pain behavior was I felt like I owed the people who were taking care of me. I felt indebtedness to them. Here's where I had to remember, again, that on down the line after I would be off the drugs and through the pain program, I would be able to do lots of things for myself and for them. In any case, they really didn't think of it as a debt. It was all in my mind. I was their family and what they did for me they did out of love, not because they expected me to do something for them. When I was in so much pain and on medication I didn't see things quite clearly.

I had to keep the lines of communication open. That was very important. Granted, it was hard for me, but it still had to be done. Communication is vital. It was important to open up and express how I felt in my relationship with family. If the lines of communication weren't kept open, we could drift apart and I could lose someone very important to me.

There were stories about marriages that couldn't withstand the stress of dealing with one partner who had chronic pain. I was concerned about my marriage and family. The only way things could work out for me was if they worked out at home, too. I needed to bring my family to the clinic on family day each Friday. It was important for my husband and children to understand what I was going through in the pain program. Otherwise, they wouldn't have had a clue as to what was really going on inside my head when I talked to them. We needed each other's support. It wasn't easy for me or my family to accept chronic pain would be with me for the rest of my life, but with God's help we would find a way.

Journal Entry, April 17, 1996

I had a tough day at the pain management clinic. I was one of the patients to break down and cry in class about having chronic pain. At times, this is all quite overwhelming. It isn't easy for anyone in the group. I need all the help I can get. I'm fighting for my life and future.

I won't be able to just go to the class and get well, as I had hoped. It takes more than that. I'll never be the person I was before...I've accepted that fact, but has my family accepted how I'm going to be for the rest of my life? Will they still want me? I try not to worry about things I can't control, but that's nearly impossible. I am a natural born worrier.

I just don't know how things will turn out, but I do think I'll be a better person for having gone through this experience and survived. For some reason, I'll probably never know, God wants me to feel this pain.

I'm continuing to write in my journal about my experiences. People have always said, "Write about something you know." Well, whether I want to or not, I'm getting to be an expert on chronic pain. It's my life. Is this what God wants me to do? Maybe, in time, I can help other people understand chronic pain. Something positive has to come out of all this misery.

The only thing is I don't want to lose my family because of all my problems. Somehow, I will have to come to some kind of understanding about all these feelings. God, please help me stand the pain without the drugs and let things be all right with my family.

The number one thing to remember when going through the program was that I was getting off the drugs and there would be dark times before growth. I was fighting my way back to find myself. This was something I had to do for myself. I had to hang in there and follow through on what I had learned. I couldn't let anything get in the way of my goal, not even my family. I understand it was my life and choice as to how I wanted to live it. The pain could control me or I could take back control of my life. The responsibility was entirely mine.

Coming down off the drugs was a new experience. Sometimes I had so many emotions built up I couldn't express them all. I'd been in a zombie state for so long it was hard to start opening up again. It took time to rediscover the person I used to be before I started taking the prescription drugs. The real person was buried inside, screaming to get out, maybe not physically but emotionally.

A big part of the process was learning how to deal with things I hadn't dealt with before. Things were brought up that I tended to keep at the back of my mind. For instance, that this chronic pain was forever. I had to bring this out into the light and examine it in order to face reality. I had to accept the fact the pain would always be with me. I had to face my relationship with loved ones. I had to deal with reality, not the drug state I'd been living in. It was time to face the music, I could do it one step at a time. If I tripped, I'd have to pick myself up, dust myself off and start again.

Pain behavior is an important concept. People will be using this term to describe what's going on with chronic pain patients for a long time to come. Since the beginning of time people have had pain. They've tried to figure out why they have it and they've tried to measure it. There are all sorts of ways they've tried to do this.

A general example could be by putting one's hand in an ice bucket and seeing how long they could stand it. They've tried to measure it by what was called "self-report." It was where I would rate myself or my pain on a scale of one to ten. There are problems of trying to measure pain this way because nobody else knows what I mean. Everybody's definition of what intolerable pain means is different. Physicians have been mostly unsuccessful at measuring pain. Not because a lot of effort hasn't been put into it, but because pain cannot easily be measured. It is an internal perception, meaning only the patient has access to it. It doesn't register on any device known to mankind.

Don't let anybody tell you they've measured your pain because they can't do it. The MRI is the most sophisticated diagnostic device we have, and it shows zero about pain; mine or anyone else's.

I could go out to any mall in the country and take a random bunch of people and do MRI's on all of them. I could give each one of them a questionnaire about pain symptoms and intensity and guess what I would find? Some people would have horrible MRI's with bulging disc, pinched nerves, and have no pain. Then there would be other people who with perfectly normal MRI's have lots of pain. Isn't that interesting? What would I conclude? Nobody's going to tell me how much pain I have based on an MRI as this wonderful high tech equipment can only tell the doctors about structural problems which structural problems do not always equal pain.

My neurologist told me back in the heyday of neurosurgery they used to cut people up when they came in and said, "My back hurts." They would do ten or twelve surgeries to try to fix the problem. They don't do it like that anymore, because they know surgery isn't always the answer.

Physicians have gotten very frustrated because they can't measure pain. When they can measure anger, that will be the day they can measure pain. This was what the psychologists call "Constra." This is the word meaning "an internal state." Think of pain as an internal feeling. Only the individual who has the pain has access to the degree of pain.

As I stated earlier, some very smart people, (one of them a psychologist named Wilburn Fordyce), came up with the idea of Pain Behavior. Defined simply, pain behavior is any behavior that indicates to another person I have pain. Any behavior I do that signals or lets someone else know I am in pain, is my pain behavior.

Pain behavior is usually divided into verbal and nonverbal actions. Examples of my nonverbal pain behavior was using a cane, limping, holding my arm, taking medication, or wearing a back brace. The way I stood, walked, or sat in the doctor's office showed signs of nonverbal pain behavior.

My pain behavior could be measured. They watched me at the clinic, and when I limped or rubbed my back they got the idea I was in pain. They video taped me and showed me things I was doing that I wasn't even aware of. People can be trained to stop showing signs of pain. They did this with me and it changed my life, because it changed the way people reacted to me.

An example of verbal pain behavior was me talking about my pain, often initiated by someone asking me, how did I sleep last night? When did I have surgery? How long had I been taking narcotics? And then there were the ones where I said, "Oh, I hurt all the time." Or if someone video taped me while I made the bed and I said, "Well, I'm not very good at this. When I get down on my hands and knees, I can't get back up." Or I said, "Oh gees, this hurts so bad." These were examples of verbal pain behavior.

Pain behaviors can actually be counted. Let's say in the initial three minutes before I had treatment, I had forty nonverbal pain behaviors and sixty verbal pain behaviors. Then I had some treatment that was supposed to affect pain. Whatever it was a spinal block or nerve block, anything to help the pain. Then they re-video taped me and noted twelve verbal pain behaviors and sixteen nonverbal pain behaviors. Noticing an incredible drop in pain behavior, this showed I was getting better. The treatment had helped and my family and friends were noticing a difference in me. They were actually saying, "You look better."

Fordyce said, "Now we have a way to measure pain." This was an enormous step. The second thing he came up with was the theory that there are two causes of pain. One was obvious as when I saw someone limping, because of a physical pain. The second was not quite so obvious. The second cause of pain behavior was *Habit.*

The type of injury could predict the type of pain. For example, pain in the first year after a car accident would be 100% physical pain. It would be zero percent for habit, because the person had not had any opportunity to learn pain behavior.

Yet, if pain continues well past the first year, there is a huge influence of pain behavior "habits" which literally keep the pain alive and unless one can acknowledge these behaviors, the pain will not easily go away.

Any habit strengthens over time. In six months to a year-and-a-half, I had developed some pretty bad habits when it came to pain. The thing was I wasn't aware this had happened to me until the people at the pain clinic brought it to my attention. And those bad habits were difficult to break.

Most habits are learned over time; whether it's yelling at my kids, avoiding conflict, or whatever. I engaged in a behavior and immediately after the behavior there was a reward. When this happened, the probability of the behavior went up because of the reinforcement with the reward.

When I went to the circus and saw the bears ride the bicycles around, those bears had learned the behavior and were rewarded for it by getting treats. Their behavior had been shaped. The behavior was under the control of the rewards. If the trainers didn't feed the bears, they wouldn't ride those bicycles anymore.

Learning is a very powerful thing. Rewards are much more powerful than punishment. If I tried to get people to do things by punishment, there would be all sorts of problems.

Pain behavior does not equal pain. Most people have a difficult time with this concept. Pain and pain behavior are separate things. My pain behavior was any signals to others that I was in pain and it brought me attention. It became a habit over time. It was a common situation for people to ask about my pain and I had to sit my loved ones down and tell them to help me not to focus on my pain. This was a way they could really help me. When I got up in the morning, I wanted them not to ask about my back. If I wanted to tell them about it, I would, but preferred they didn't bring it up. This made it a lot easier for me not to focus on my pain.

Most people cared about me and they would be good for a couple of days and then they'd slip and ask, "How's your back?" They were like me, in the habit of asking when they saw me in pain. I had to gently remind them of the talk we had. I said, "I know you love me and care about me but I need you to try to help me by not focusing on my pain, unless, I want to talk to you about it. It's hard for me and I know it's hard for you, too." After awhile, even the thickest person can unlearn behaviors, myself included.

If it was reinforced enough, then the behavior would have continued and increased. Attention was the reward for my pain behavior. Remember, reward has tremendous effect on behavior. When I reversed the contingencies, it was a big responsibility. Anything that was this powerful I could easily misuse, if I wasn't careful. I had to caution myself when I was working with behavioral modification. If I was assertive to people, "Well, here's the problem, every time I start talking you interrupt me. I want you to stop doing this." I had to tell people what I wanted. Re-enforcers were chosen by the ability to influence behavior. A million dollars would be a great enforcer.

The point is, pain behavior comes under the same laws of learning, whether I liked it or not. Whether the people in my life were aware of it or whether I was aware of it, these laws applied.

My verbal and nonverbal pain behavior had some habit components. They may have been very tiny, but they were there. There were some things I could change if I watched myself. I could inform people in my environment I didn't want to focus on my pain. It would take care of itself as my pain behavior decreased. This happened as I felt better physically.

What I did in the program with all verbal pain behavior was pretend like it wasn't happening. Not because I didn't hear well or I was insensitive, but because I knew, and I believed this was happening and I was doing myself and my fellow students a great favor by not participating in future learning of pain behavior. I didn't want that for myself or anyone else.

When I first came into the program, pain was my life. It was where I was focused. As time went by, I learned not to focus on the pain and instead regain control of my life. I'd been to the edge and back, and I was winning.

JULIE'S SUCCESS STORY

Treating Failed Back Syndrome Pain

"I spent 98% percent of my time in a wheelchair or using a cane. And I could only sleep in fifteen to twenty minute catnaps. That kind of pain really wears you down. Now, the way I feel can't be said on paper—it's that much better. I'm off the pain medication. I'm back to work again. I can even do my own housework."

—Julie

When she was forty-two, Julie slipped at work and landed backwards on her buttocks, causing a back injury. After her injury, she developed pain shooting down her right leg, which her doctor diagnosed as sciatica.

Julie was initially sent to a spine surgeon for a possible fusion. The surgeon determined she did not need a fusion, but did perform a nerve block and a discogram with an anesthetic solution. After these procedures, Julie felt 50% pain relief. She also tried physical therapy, but it did not relieve her pain. She also took a combination of pain medications, antidepressants, and anti-inflammatory drugs, none of which were effective in relieving her pain.

About one year after her injury, Julie was evaluated for Advanced Pain Therapy Neurostimulation. She underwent a screening test using a temporary lead, a special medical wire, placed at the area of the spine that corresponded with where she felt pain. She experienced pain relief in one leg—but her low back and right buttock areas were not improved. These results suggested using a neurostimulation system with two leads, and this gave Julie pain relief in her leg, buttocks, and lower back.

At first, Julie could only spend three minutes on a treadmill just after surgery, but within three weeks she had increased her workout to three miles.

Since receiving Advanced Pain Therapy Neurostimulation, Julie has experienced 100% pain relief. She has continued to take an anti-inflammatory drug, but no longer takes other pain medications and has returned to work, but stays away from duties which require her to sit for long periods of time.

Will I feel the Neurostimulation system inside me, and will people notice?

The IPG, internal battery, nor receiver make any noise. It may be felt as a small bulge under your skin and it does not normally show through your clothes. The device is about 2.25 inches, 6 cm wide, 2 inches, 5.2 cm high, and one-half inch, 1 cm thick. It is usually implanted in the lower abdomen where it is most comfortable and least visible. You can discuss placement with your doctor before surgery and decide the best location for the IPG or receiver. If your doctor recommends a radio frequency system, the transmitter will be visible and is usually worn on the belt like a pager. In addition, an antenna must be placed on your skin for the system to work.

CHAPTER ELEVEN

Personal Responsibility and Self Help

"When you were born, you cried and the world rejoiced. Live your life in such a manner that when you die the world cries and you rejoice." *-Unknown Native American*

I had to accept there isn't a cure for Chronic Pain Syndrome. There isn't any magic potion. The best I would be able to do was to learn skills that would help me better manage this problem, to help me get my life back on track. I'd be able to do things I wanted to do and not be depressed, not be angry, and not be anxious despite having a disability.

Previously, I had a history of viewing my problem of chronic pain from a perspective not useful to me. I wouldn't have been sitting in a pain management program if the medical model had worked. I would have been cured.

I've discussed earlier, that I'd been raised on what was called a medical model. The medical model simply meant when a person got injured they went to the expert doctors and got a diagnosis. This would tell them why they were having problems from a physical standpoint. Along with those tests, they would have pain. There were all sorts of wonderful diagnostic tests out there, which most of us have had. Most people have had MRIs, Cat Scans, EEGs, etc. Of course X-rays are one of the common ones. Some people have had other really painful diagnostic procedures. I went to the experts and they did all those things to me. The purpose of those diagnostic techniques was to find out why I had my problem with pain.

In the medical model, here is how the thinking goes. If there is something wrong with someone physically, it often manifests itself in pain. There is a reason for this system. Pain is a symptom. A symptom really meant an outside manifestation of an inside problem. When I had pain, medical people believed me because there was something wrong with my body. Those tests were an attempt to find out what was wrong. It was strictly physical. Yet all those diagnostic tests were purely physical and extremely limited.

For instance, an MRI showed nothing about muscle or tendon problems. Although most of us with chronic pain have serious muscular problems, it showed nothing on the MRI. However, I put great stock in those tests by virtue of how many people have had them. Based on this, I got a diagnosis which was supposed to tell the world what was wrong with me, then the treatment was selected from there and was supposed to fix my problem.

In this medical model everybody lives happily ever after and I am cured. This was what I had been taught throughout my lifetime. It had been burned into my brain. No matter what happened to me, at one time, I thought the doctors could still fix me. I was wrong.

I read about this high tech stuff in the newspaper all the time. In today's society, I highly value medicine; not just medicine, but high-tech, expensive medicine. This is no longer a society of home remedies. I was bombarded with this day and night through the TV and newspapers.

The medical model said, "If there was something wrong with me physically those experts ought to find it and be able to fix it. That is your God-given right."

The whole issue with health care is that most people with medical coverage believe anybody ought to be able to walk into any health care provider with any problem and get it fixed. Unfortunately, it just isn't so. There are millions of people to prove the medical model wrong, for instance, the eighty-six million of us diagnosed with Chronic Pain Syndrome.

Journal Entry, April 25, 1996

I had a good day at class. I'm in a good mood. I'm still having a hard time giving up on a cure, or the medical model, as they like to call it. However, my eyes have been opened and I have no excuses, but to believe this new truth I've been taught. I'm doing much better. The pain is still with me, but now it's different. I control it instead of it controlling me. I'm winning the battle!

This class is a stepping stone for those of us with chronic pain. They have given me the tools to deal with living with this disorder. Now, what I do with my future is up to me.

Each and every student in my class has been there for each of us at one time or another, whether it was with a hug or a pat on the shoulder. We are always there for each other when it counts.

It's hard to understand this phenomenon unless you are living with it on a daily basis. Yet it has created an unbreakable bond among our support group. I will never forget these people who helped me to grow and accept my challenges in life.

The basic belief when coming into a program with the medical model is that the patient plays a passive role. The stereotypical medical intervention or treatment is usually surgery. Many people have had major surgery but don't really understand what the surgery was about or what the surgeon was doing.

For instance, let's talk about a common medical emergency, which is not an injury...let's say Joe had acute appendicitis. He woke up with the most awful stomach ache he'd ever had in his entire life, couldn't straighten up, and felt like he was going to die and ended up going to the Emergency Room in excruciating pain.

The ER physician did the diagnostic test by simply feeling his abdomen and muscles. He said, "Oh my God, it's an urgent situation, your appendix is about to burst. We have to take you right up to the operating room. We have to get your appendix out."

Most people wouldn't know their appendix from a bicycle wheel, so Joe said, "Fine, do anything to get rid of this pain." They knocked him out and took out his appendix. He assumed they took out the right thing but he wouldn't know if they didn't. They could've said they took it out, and took out something else for all he knew. However, Joe had faith that they did do what they said they would do. He'd been taught to have great faith in doctors and medicine. He woke up and was kind of groggy since they had given him some kind of medication. Of course, the treatment was the operation. After a while, he was good as new. His role, as they used to say on the Greyhound Bus commercial was, "Leave the driving to us."

A lot of people have no knowledge of what is happening to their body, or of what the medical community is doing to them. People with chronic pain become exceptions because we are angry and frustrated with our pain. We've learned to lose faith because of the pain we've been going through and the failure of the medical model to cure that pain.

Before chronic pain, I was a passive patient who didn't have any knowledge of what decisions were being made for me and I was a common example. If you don't believe this, just go to any hospital and observe the patients. Most would do anything the doctor or nurse told them to, without giving it a second thought.

Medication errors aren't only due to the professionals coming in with the wrong medication, but with the patient taking the wrong medication. For instance, I'd been taking two brown pills and a white one for three weeks. The nurse came in with three blue ones and a green one and I would take them without even questioning her. They happened to be for the person in bed B and I was in bed A, but I would take them anyway. Some of us check our brain at the door when we go into a hospital.

With this medical model background, you can imagine how difficult it was for me to maneuver through chronic pain. This model had failed me.

As I stated earlier, people love the medical model. It was still hard for me to give it up. It had quite the attraction. There was a cure for the medical model, but not for us folks with chronic pain. The biggest attraction was the doctors, the experts who were responsible for the medical model. If something went wrong I could say, "That darned doctor didn't do the right thing for me. He got paid all that money and put me through so much pain and nothing has changed. I still have constant, excruciating pain." People are usually furious with doctors by the time they enter a program like the Pikes Peak Pain program. Everyone had their "doctor story" to tell.

It was a fairly external point of view. The promise of the medical model was that I could be a passive person and someone would take care of me. The responsibility was out there somewhere. As a patient, would have very little responsibility in the medical model. I basically would do what I was told to do. It was like being in the Army. "Take two of these before bed time," the doctor said. I couldn't read the written prescription anyway. It would've been unusual if I would've asked, "So what are these?"

The doctor would answer, "Well, they are pain pills."

"Are there any side effects?"

"Minimal," he would say.

"How long do I have to take them?"

"Well, we'll just try them out and see how you do."

"Are these going to interact with any of the other drugs I'm taking?"

"No."

The answers would be fairly straightforward and seemingly factual because they were coming from on high. The unsaid message was to hurry up and finish with your questioning.

The model is still able to accommodate a clear, medical and acute problem and it will work well for that. If I ever had to have bypass heart surgery, I would thank my lucky stars somebody came up with the operation. Not only would it save my life, but I would feel better than I did before I had it.

Even after getting through the Pikes Peak Pain program, I will not be cured. What I will learn are ways of dealing with the issues of having chronic pain. When I became clear with this point, I will have come a long way. To accept I would have to live with chronic pain for the rest of my life was a great challenge in itself.

Usually, it would take a person a long time to unlearn the medical model. They would go to the Mayo Clinic or anywhere they could to try to find a cure, only to find out there is no cure. The goal of the pain program was to get me to my best possible shape physically, socially, psychologically, and vocationally with the maximum medical improvement.

When entering the pain program, some people diagnosed with chronic pain were frightened to death...like me. They were scared of the future. It was a reasonable fear. I was frightened and I needed to put that fear to work for me, not against me. I converted fear into energy or motivation to learn as much as I could with the time I had in the program.

However I felt, or whatever skills I'd learn, which I could apply and improve upon, was all I was going to get. There was no where else to go from here, so I had to make the most of the program.

Those who had done well with the program, that had improved physically, did their exercises and applied all the things they learned. If they chose to go back to work, it wasn't an unreasonable goal, although it might not have been the same job they'd had, especially if it was a real physically demanding one.

About 50% of the Pikes Peak Pain program patients were able to go back to work in some capacity. The other 50% that weren't able were mostly due to other health reasons associated with the chronic pain.

Here are the odds without any intervention: If a person has a back, neck, or shoulder injury and has been out of work for a year or more, the probability of ever returning to work in their natural life is two in five. The goal of the pain program was to increase the odds.

Whether they could make a difference for me, they didn't know. It wasn't up to them. It was up to me and my own situation, my body, and my particular health problem. It was my responsibility and it depended on how much I wanted to get better.

I can't stress it enough. It was a lost cause to continue to search for the magic potion to cure me. There was no cure and I could only get better when I finally accepted that. Once I gave it up, then I was able to shift to the self help model. I knew about this model because before chronic pain, I'd applied it almost every day in my own life as a consumer.

A self help model takes the person who has a stake in the problem and educates that person, waking them up and imparting knowledge so they are no longer ignorant. I thought of some of the stuff I did when I was sixteen. I didn't know how I survived it all. Back then I was ignorant, now I know better. I have more knowledge, so I don't do things like I did at that time.

The goal of the pain program was to educate me. Some of it was upsetting. I didn't like hearing about a lot of things, but I needed to know about them.

Actually, the self help model I learned about showed me that I had a rehabilitation problem, not a medical one. I was *disabled* because of the pain. I didn't like this term. Physically challenged sounded better to me.

Fortunately, the goal of the pain program was to help me learn that while I would forever have this life-changing disability, the effects of this problem on my life could, and would, be minimized with intervention. I would learn to behave in a different manner by the time I completed the program...I'd be able to do more, enjoy my life more, and hopefully get back to work. The icing on the cake would be that my family should be able to enjoy me more as I grew less depressed and they were able to feel less conflicted.

The staff were my teachers and they were teaching me how to live with chronic pain. Every once in a while they'd slip and call themselves therapist or medical counselors, but they were my teachers. They weren't fixating on medical stuff. I was learning a new lifestyle. When I learned well enough, then and only then would I be able to change my life for the good.

CHAPTER TWELVE

Communication Skills and Chronic Pain

"For it is important that awake people be awake, or a breaking line may discourage them back to sleep; the signals we give—yes or no, or maybe—should be clear: the darkness around us is deep." *- William Stafford*

Communication skills are important to all of us, but for those living in a world of anxiety, stress, depression, and oftentimes anger...communication skills are key in getting along with others and getting along with pain. With this in mind, it's easy to understand why I needed to send to others around me, clear and precise information about the pain I was experiencing and exactly what, if anything, I wanted others to help me with during theses tough moments. If I couldn't do this well, I could get into a lot of trouble...both physically and emotionally.

While I wasn't as young as I used to be, I was as young as I'd like to be and I knew that my goal was to have the best possible life while managing the pain that lived around my neck like dead weight. I knew that in order to master this beast, I would have to stay focused every single day and learn as much as I could about my options. For me, knowledge was my new power.

Journal Entry, May 8, 1996

Today we talked about goals and learning different ways of communication skills. One thing we talked about was sending and receiving information. The main thing is to be able to send clear information and be able to really listen when someone is talking to me.

Not many of us really listen. A lot of time as the person is speaking to you, you're already judging them. If I spend all my time judging people I won't have time to love them.

This gave me a lot to think about. I always thought I was a good listener, now I'm not sure. There are many things I have to consider when I'm communicating with my loved ones. I don't want to be too assertive, but I don't want to be a doormat either. I'll have to work on this and find the middle ground.

Being assertive is a much misunderstood term, as oftentimes people think being assertive is the same thing as being aggressive. Far from the truth. Being assertive is a communication skill that allows us to make our needs known, without harming others in the process. Being aggressive can sometimes go beyond simple assertiveness, and can cross the boundaries of other people to achieve the desired results. An aggressive person can easily mow others over in their quest for what they want while an assertive person can accomplish meeting their needs without causing harm or injury along the way.

While growing up, I had been taught not to be either aggressive or assertive...the two were somehow seen as the same thing. The result was that even as a grown up I had a hard time making my needs known and frequently I simply sat like a bump on a log while others around me got their way, as I sat silently resentful of the results.

On my journey I began to learn that being assertive was a skill like many others, and as such, could be learned, even at this late date in my life. Learning to say and do what I wanted to say and do took time and practice. First of all I had to know exactly what it was I wanted, then what my opinions were about the situation, what was important to me, and what my needs and desires were. Most importantly, I had to better understand myself.

If I said, "Let's go out to lunch, what do you like to eat?" You either have an opinion or you don't. You either don't care or you have a strong preference.

An example would be, let's say I wanted Chinese food, and felt strongly about it. I already knew where I wanted to go. Now, the second part was communicating to others where I want to go for lunch. There are two parts, one meant knowing what I wanted, what I wanted to do, what I wanted to say, and what was important to me. The second part is communicating my wishes to others.

What usually happened was that I, the one who wanted Chinese food, would just sit there and let someone else decide where we would go for lunch. I told myself I didn't want to be too pushy or rude so I ended up going where everyone else wanted to go. It was sort of like, "You go first," "No, you go first." "I'll take the check," "No, I'll take the check." This is a mundane example, but most assertiveness concerns involve not sending clear signals. If I couldn't be assertive about something as small as lunch, how could I make my needs known to my husband, kids, or friends. This is a simple thing and most people just sit there because they'd been taught to be polite. They always put themselves second or third or one hundred. They just wait. I realized I was like that and needed to learn a new way of life. I started developing assertiveness in small ways.

When someone said, "Let's go eat Mexican food" I had to look inside my head and heart and I realized I hated Mexican food. I knew two things. I loved Chinese food and I was really in the mood for it and I hated Mexican food. If nothing happened, I knew where I was going to end up eating lunch. I was going to have Mexican food.

What it's all about is personal choice. It isn't better to like Chinese or Mexican, as a matter of fact who cares? It was a matter of preference. Almost everything I talk about or discuss is a matter of opinion. My opinion. And it's important I learn to communicate it.

What I am suggesting is it isn't a whole lot different whether I liked Chinese food or Mexican food, maybe a little bit more important, but not a whole lot. So I started there and gave myself permission to have divergent opinions. Those are different opinions because everybody is different, everybody is special. It would be an extremely boring world if we were all alike.

So I started there. Unassertiveness was a problem I had some of the time. It was my failure to choose, however, it wasn't a legitimate failure to choose, it was me talking myself out of something I preferred or making excuses. Basically I would chicken out. I would lose my nerve. I said to myself, "The next time we have that discussion I'll be darned if I'm going to eat Mexican food, it makes me barf." Then I would go along with all my friends and wanting to please them, and all those reasons I had to be assertive would go right out the window. Someone said, "Wasn't it neat when we went to Dos Hombres? Let's go to Dos Hombres, again." If I didn't say anything, I'd failed to exercise my option, which was to state my opinion. That's all I'm talking about. I wasn't talking about bossing people around, putting pressure on them, hurting their feelings, or making them feel uncomfortable. I was merely sending a piece of information that happened to be my opinion. Just communicating by getting my point across that I would rather go eat Chinese food.

I needed to keep it that simple or else I'd get all tangled up in what the skill was. The purpose of this skill's goal is not to get my way, but to clearly communicate what I desired or needed. Once I'd done that, it was all over. I only had control over one person's behavior, and that was my own. I could make it perfectly clear where I would like to go to eat Chinese food. Then I could try to be assertive and add all those reasons why I wanted to go there and try to influence the others to go with me. Then I said, "Do you want to go?" They said, "If you want to eat lunch alone you can go eat Chinese food, but we want to go to Dos Hombres." Now, I had another choice. This was the problem most of us have some of the time. I knew what I wanted. I knew what I wanted to do. I knew what my opinion was but I didn't do or say anything about it, because I wanted to go with my friends.

Another problem with assertiveness is the thought or belief that people can actually make others do things by ordering them around or threatening them. That wouldn't be effective for me. Unfortunately, this is the way of a lot of families. For instance, they try to tell the person they should believe in God and if they don't believe, they'll go to Hell. It wasn't stated as an opinion. They were trying to force their opinions on that person.

There is nothing wrong with having strong opinions, but I needed to realize that was all they were, only opinions. Even extreme beliefs of religion or politics, are not facts. They are opinions.

The bottom line was, I needed to learn to choose for myself. It was simple; I looked inside and decided what I wanted to do or say and said or did what I wanted to do. It was learning to stand up for myself. I needed to be clear with what I wanted or said. Sometimes people will jump back and forth from non-assertiveness to over-assertiveness. I had two behaviors, I either had non-assertiveness, where I didn't say or do anything, or I went along with whatever happened, or I was over-assertive where I was trying to make people do stuff or manipulate them to get what I wanted.

"Well, why don't you want to go to that movie?" I could have said.

"I don't like all that blood and violence. Thanks, but I don't care to go."

"I think you're hung up about this kind of movie and this would probably be therapeutic for you."

"Look, I just don't want to go."

"You know, I think you probably need professional help with this," I could have insisted.

If I would've said all that to someone, all totally uncalled for, I would have crossed the line. I could always tell when I'd crossed the line into aggressiveness. It was when I was really applying pressure to get what I wanted.

Being unassertive is the easiest path to follow with the least resistance for the short run. I believed if I didn't say or do anything, I was safe. It was like being convinced all of my sins were sins of omission. I wasn't there, I didn't do anything. I didn't say anything. I didn't know what happened. I'd learned this at a young age. As a child, I was systematically taught to be non-assertive.

An assertive exchange was simply when I stated my own opinion or desire. I told the person what I desired and then I might have told them the consequences of what they decided to do about the situation. This was all clean. It only got dirty when I stepped out of the realm of clear opinions. I knew all this through my work. When I was working on location, the director would tell me exactly what was expected of me for each take.

If I didn't do what was expected I might not like being told or criticized about it, especially if I was sensitive to criticism. But at least I didn't live in a crazy world where they saved up all my mistakes for six months or so and unloaded on me or lead me to losing my job. It was somewhat upsetting in the short run to be told of my mistakes on my job performance, but to save it up for six months or so would be downright cruel. It works better to know your mistakes up front.

People who are non-assertive tend to label those who are assertive as being aggressive. Why? Because we aren't used to people being direct. I can be direct and kind with someone and they will be sort of blown away, because they aren't used to people calling them on their mistakes.

A lot of people have learned to use crummy interpersonal behavior with their family. Then they get out in the real world and this is totally unacceptable in a work setting. It's important to remember there's a fine line between assertiveness and aggressiveness.

The more personal responsibility I have, the more control I have in my life. The more I take charge of my life, the more I discover a deeper sense of who I am. The only voice that matters is the one inside my head.

FRANK'S SUCCESS STORY

Treating Pain Due to
Compression Fractures from Osteoporosis

The first sign that something was wrong came one day when Frank bent over and felt a stab of pain in his lower back. Over-the-counter ointment, heat, and a massage from his wife, Mae, helped Frank feel better. But unknown to himself or anyone else at the time, osteoporosis—a destructive bone disorder—was wearing away bits of his spine.

One day, Frank was getting up from a chair when pain hit him harder than ever. An x-ray showed that he had suffered a compression fracture in his lower spine. The pain was unbearable. Frank rated it a ten on a pain scale of one to ten. He received oxycodone with acetaminophen, percocet, and steroid injection for the intense pain. The relief, however, was only temporary.

In the months that followed, Frank's pain increased substantially. Emergency room visits, steroid injections, and prescribed combinations of morphine sulfate, MS contim, oxycodone with acetaminophen, tylox, propoxiphene, and darvocet moderately relieved his pain, but Frank's discomfort was constant.

"The pain medication would wear off fast, and I could only give him a dose every four hours," said Mae, remembering the suffering her husband went through. "It was terrible for us to see him in so much pain and not be able to help."

After minimal pain relief from oxycodone hydrochloride controlled-release tablets, oxycontin, hydromophone, dilauded, and transcutaneous electrical nerve stimulation, TENS, and anesthesiologist specializing in pain management told Frank about Medtronic Advanced Pain Therapy Intrathecal. The therapy had been successful with other patients with chronic pain. Frank was interested.

Two weeks after a successful screening test, Frank underwent surgery to begin APT Intrathecal. He experienced no complications, and went home the day following the procedure.

Frank's pain decreased about 50% at first, and continued to decline over the following months. He now rates his pain as only one to two on a ten point scale. "The pain is nearly gone for me," Frank said.

Frank had experienced no side effects from the therapy. With APT Intrathecal, pain no longer controls Frank's life.

"This pump made all the difference in the world for me," Frank said. "I had pain on and off for a long time, and sometimes it was terrible. Now, it doesn't bother me at all. As far as my back is concerned, I feel as good as ever."

How will I know when the pump needs to be replaced?

Your doctor or nurse will be able to tell you the state of the battery when he or she checks the pump with the programmer during your regular refill appointment. In addition, the battery in the pump has a built-in alarm to let you know when it needs to be replaced. The pump emits a soft, high pitched beeping sound repeated several times per minute. If you hear the alarm sound, call your doctor immediately. Some people are unable to hear the alarm, so it is important to notify your doctor if you notice a change in pain relief or other changes as well.

CHAPTER THIRTEEN

Conflict Management and Chronic Pain

"And should this not be of importance, since not until a man is finished with the future can he be entirely and undividedly in the present?" *-Soren Kierkegaard*

Conflict is something all of us have and will have our whole life and it will never be eliminated. Other patients in the clinic often talked about going places to eliminate their conflict. It couldn't be done. I'd have to lead an extremely boring life if this were to happen. Everything would be perfect. People would have to agree with everything I said and did. There was a fat chance of that happening. And if I did manage to limit all conflict from my life, what would I learn? I wouldn't learn anything. I'd still hold all the opinions I held when I was sixteen, when I knew everything. I'd stop growing.

Most people hate conflict, which usually involves a disagreement of some kind and is inevitable when dealing with people. Usually, the conflict will arise over an opinion not based on fact. Most conflict is an emotional thing and people are afraid of being hurt and in our society, people aren't good at dealing with conflict. In other societies, it is much more acceptable to disagree or yell and scream.

When a conflict arises I learned it should be a matter of trusting myself. I'd done something my whole life with managing conflict. Day in and day out, week in week out, I'd managed my own conflict. Maybe I hadn't done it very well at times, but I had managed my own personal conflict. The question was one of management, not one of elimination.

I came from a family where disagreement or conflict wasn't tolerated and I was shy. This isn't uncommon. We each have different learning histories. Nothing can change that. I am who I am, now. Regimented from my birth, I am the total measure of what I have learned. My point is that I can learn something different. I can change. It's difficult, but if I couldn't change the way I managed my conflict, this wouldn't have had any meaning for me.

If I thought I was some kind of fixed product because of the traits I had, then I was wrong. "I'm not a big believer in traits. I'm helpless. I'm introverted. I keep to myself because I'm uncomfortable expressing my feelings."

"Was I happy with that?"

If I would have said, "Yeah I am," then that would have been the end of the story."

If I would say instead, "No, not really, I'm unhappy to be like this, it's starting to give me ulcers. My marriage is on the rocks and I can't keep any friends," then things could be different. I could change because I wasn't an introvert. I was a person who had learned behaviors that made me appear to be an introvert but I was really only a person who resisted change.

This is another skill I learned. To start with, I sometimes became upset because of a difference of opinion. I hated any kind of arguing, especially with someone close to me that I cared about. It was even more difficult when there was a long history with the person. I realized I couldn't eliminate disagreement. I had to agree on a certain number of things. The second thing I had to agree upon was that all conflict was not necessarily bad. This was sometimes difficult for me to accept. I knew that intellectually, but emotionally it was hard to grasp. I hated conflict because I was concerned about being tricked or getting hurt.

Journal Entry, May 11, 1996
Today, I feel scattered and had a hard time coping. The kids were fighting about something and I didn't have the strength to

contend with it. I love them with all my heart, but right now I have to take care of myself. If I get involved in the disagreement I'll be useless the rest of the day.

When I get upset it makes me hurt more. I can't handle much stress at this time in my life. It causes me to hurt so bad. I went to bed early tonight because I was mentally tired and physically worn out. Rob settled the argument between the kids. I don't know what I'd do without him. Thank God for my wonderful husband.

Most conflicts don't escalate beyond words. While sticks and stones can break my bones, words can never hurt me. Nobody ever died from words. If I allow words to cause me stress, that leads to increased muscle tension and this causes my pain to intensify.

When I'm having a bad time emotionally I can see it in my body. How well I manage conflict affects how I physically feel. The good thing about this is once I became aware of it, I could learn how to manage my personal conflict and I got better with handling it in time.

To me, most conflict was an emotional thing and I was afraid of being hurt. This was especially true with my personal relationships. I was afraid to say what I really meant because I might lose my special someone. My biggest fear was being left alone with my pain in a nursing home. Yet if I didn't open up and share my feelings with my husband, the situation would fester and get worse as time went by, until all lines of communication were cut off and there wasn't anything left.

Other people weren't responsible for how I felt. I had to take control of my emotions and open up to let them know. They weren't mind readers. While it was hard work to overcome the fear of rejection, I built my skills step by step.

The most common conflict management strategy is avoidance. Some people will pretend the incident didn't happen in order not to participate. That's okay. One of the most usual forms of conflict is when one person who is upset with another person will talk about the first person in a negative manner to a group of other people. They will avoid confrontation because of fear, but they want everyone else to know what a butthead the other person is.

There are ways to ignore conflict; like walking away, claming up and not talking about the incident, blowing up at the other person, pouting, take ten before you speak, drinking or using drugs, watching TV, sleeping or eating. The alternative is to approach the conflict head on. This is the best way for me, so I can get it out of my system and move on with my life.

A negative example would be if I was driving down the roadway and someone cut me off. I might start calling the person names and shake my fist at them. By this time, I'm really upset and this causes me stress, which causes muscle tension, which causes me more pain. The person who cut me off may not even know he cut me off or just ignored me and went on his way, not even giving the incident a second thought. By the time I get to work and am still dwelling on the situation which makes me more frustrated, I actually internalize this conflict and cause harm to my body. The bigger question is, "Is it worth it?"

Because the other driver was a jerk, I didn't have to turn into one, too. This was where I could take control of the situation and go on and say to myself, "It's okay, just let the idiot go his way. He will get what's coming to him by someone else." It wouldn't do me any good to yell and scream at the person or run them down. It would only cause me more stress, which would cause me more pain.

I had to learn when to let go of things to avoid the stress in situations like this. If it saved me pain, then I would do what ever I needed to do. I had to let go of my anger.

Someone once said to me, "Don't sweat the small stuff, and it's all small stuff." At the time, I didn't get it, but now that I have chronic pain I can relate to it very well. I have to put my health before my anger or conflict in my life. The reality of the situation is that most people want conflict dropped. The alternative is to approach the conflict and put it behind me. This is the important part. By putting it behind me, I can get on with my life and not cause myself more internal pain.

It all depends on what situation I'm involved in as to how I should react to it. Each day I'm learning to expand my conflict management skills in ways that work for me. As with other things, I will learn and get better with it in time. Time has no meaning in the healing process. We are all unique individuals and have our own paths to follow.

CHAPTER FOURTEEN

Perfectionism and Chronic Pain

May life always bring you many reasons to smile and laugh.
— *Native American Blessing*

Those of us who have chronic pain can't do things as fast, or as long, or as many things at a time, as we used to. Many people are brought up to be perfectionist; myself included. There are a whole bunch of sayings, like "Anything worth doing, is worth doing well." I always wanted to do things well. If I didn't care about doing something well, I didn't do it. It used to be that I'd try to do everything perfectly. Yet nobody can do everything perfectly. Who was I kidding?

Journal Entry, May 26, 1996
Today was a good day. I'm having a hard time with the leg cramps at night, but by doing the stretches and exercises they are getting better. Surprise of surprises, I'm off all medication, and I'm doing OKAY.

It's good to really know what's going on around me. I'm tired of living in a fog, being dulled by the narcotics I've been taking. They told me it would take about seven months to really get the hang of what they'd been teaching me, learning to live a new lifestyle. It does take time to change, but my family can already see a difference in me and so can I. I feel good today.

The pain is with me, but I'm controlling it, instead of it controlling me. What a nice change!

One of the big things I learned this past week was that I don't have to be perfect. I know that sounds funny when I put it into words, but before chronic pain, that was how I was trying to live my life.

I'm completely happy with the Pikes Peak Pain Program. I feel like a new woman. I had to have my eyes opened about a few things. I think this program would be good for a lot of people even if they don't have chronic pain.

I'm getting excited about doing my own thing at home. Thank goodness, for this program and these people who really help people like me.

There is an alternative to living with perfectionism. I am sure, if you are a perfectionist, you wonder what I am talking about. A much more reasonable approach is to strive for excellence. Look at the difference between "I have to be perfect," and "I will strive for excellence." I think that maybe I could achieve excellence, although, I may go to my grave without an excellent performance in some areas. But I would be working hard, and that's my goal. It isn't the end state that's fueling my behavior. This is a process of striving.

To make this distinction, I use an example of athletes. There is no such thing as a perfect athlete. There is no such thing as the greatest athlete in the world, who turns in a perfect performance every time. This does not happen. They may be great, but they aren't perfect.

A lot of people think the greatest basketball player that ever lived, who is now playing again, is Michael Jordan. What was Michael Jordan's basket average? Right now, just starting over, it's about the same as everybody else. If he is so good, why doesn't he make all his shots? Well, because that's impossible, that's why. If he was a perfectionist he wouldn't be playing basketball, not for the NBA. He would have quit a long time ago. Great athletes are not perfectionists. If you think so, talk to some of them or watch an interview. Have you ever seen Michael Jordan interviewed on ESPN? They asked him, "Well, Michael, you didn't make forty points this game." He said,

"So, I'm not there to make forty points, I'm there to have a good time. I'm going to try and make as many points as I can; if I don't, I don't." Then he went and played baseball. He wasn't a perfectionist, but he was a great basketball player. He didn't need to be perfect to be great.

If I went through a list of people who had great accomplishments I'd find they didn't get that way by being a perfectionist. Tour the Olympic Training Center in Colorado Springs, Colorado and see if they use the word perfection or perfect on any of their literature or in any of their training films. They use the word excellence, but not perfectionism.

What could I do about this? I needed to change my expectations. I was a true perfectionist and I started to get nervous. True perfectionists believe they are surviving because they are perfectionistic.

I could change my expectations. A really good example is about one of my favorite contemporary poets who died recently. His name was William Stafford. He was incredibly prolific and produced a book of about two hundred poems every two months. He was absolutely amazing. When he was being interviewed they asked, "How can you write all these poems?"

He said, "I set aside time during the day and just write at this specific time."

The interviewer asked, "What happens when you're not having a good day, when creative thoughts don't come?"

You know what he said? "I lower my expectations."

That was beautiful. Because if he didn't, he wasn't going to keep writing. He was going to get frustrated and say, "God, I'm one of the best poets in America today and it's Thursday morning and I'm sitting here looking at the wall and I've got nothing but crap on my paper. I think I'll give it up and go into real estate."

That happens to a lot of perfectionist people. The impossible demand to perform perfectly leads to more stress, until the pressure becomes intolerable. The way out is to not perform. So there are a lot of perfectionists who are doing nothing. They are very unhappy because doing nothing isn't acceptable to them either.

With me having chronic pain, I could do less, or I couldn't do things as fast, or I couldn't make as much money, or I couldn't clean my house as well, or whatever. Imagine how I demanded something physically out of myself which wasn't possible for me to do. The more I demanded it, the more anxious and angry and beside myself I became. I not only demanded perfectionism from myself, I demanded it from those around me as well.

I had to remember it was all a matter of opinion. Almost everything is. If my opinion was that every human being on the face of the earth should do everything perfectly, how do you think I was going to treat the other people?

For instance, if my husband rinsed the dishes and put them in the dishwasher, but didn't bother to rinse out the sink after he was done, this would drive me crazy until I would go and do it myself. I was pretty rough on the people who meant a lot to me. Maybe I didn't really get mad, but I always picked on him because he wasn't doing things the way I liked them to be done; because he couldn't do anything right to please me.

My reactions weren't an effective way to change his behavior. The implication was he didn't do things right. Or else I would have said, "That's great, you did a wonderful job." I could have said, "When you do the dishes would you mind rinsing out the sink?" That's fine. That would've been my right. All it meant was that was the way I thought the sink should be rinsed out after the dishes were done. Of course, he could have said, "This is the way I want to do it. If you want it different, then you do it."

This could've gotten turned into a big thing because he wasn't doing things the right way for me. I could have said, "He's a slob. He's lazy, he doesn't have any standards." This could have caused a major rift in our relationship, if it was a forced issue. I liked the towels folded a certain way, the dishes had to be placed in the dishwasher a certain way, and clothes had to be folded and put in the drawers a certain way. All my coat hangers had to be the same color and face the same way. I drove my husband nuts with all this, but thank God, he loved me unconditionally.

I really had to look at this level of expectation for myself and for others. There are a lot of ways to do things which are effective. There are some ways to do certain things and if they aren't done that way significant safety or legal issues could result. I've never thought it was sensible to do things a certain way for reasons other than whether it was right or wrong, or good or bad, or the way it should be done.

What I needed to do was watch to see how much of my stress was connected to me demanding that things be done a certain way, according to my opinion. When I did, I found out I was causing a lot of unnecessary stress and more pain for myself over insignificant things.

For example, the issue of timeliness. I am a person who's quite obsessed about time. Basically, it's my judgment as to how important it is to be on time as opposed to others. I was always fifteen minutes early for appointments. As a perfectionist, there aren't enough hours in the day for me to have any time for myself. I scheduled how much time it took to vacuum my house, do my laundry, and more. It was a never ending process.

Learning to identify my perfectionistic habits, I began to recognize my intolerance for any lack of activity on my part. How often did I relax, letting it all go by, maybe laying on the couch reading a romance novel, or taking a bubble bath? Not enough. A perfectionist person doesn't have time for those things. I always had too many other important things to do.

A large percentage of people with chronic pain tend to be perfectionistic. Why? An educated guess might be because they never stop going. They go, go, go and don't take care of themselves. They try to do four things at once and they get a little bit careless. If they are in a situation where there is potential for injury, the probability of getting injured goes up.

Perfectionism was something I was doing to myself. I kept trying to go faster, even with the chronic pain, and I couldn't do it anymore. This caused depression. I had to learn to let some of it go. So what if the laundry didn't get done on Monday, finish it Tuesday and be in less pain.

It was a true learning experience. I had no choice but to take care of myself if I wanted to lead a normal life. This didn't mean to stop doing things I could still do. This meant to pace myself and let go of the, 'I have to get it done, no matter how much it hurt,' idea.

When the pain started to get more intense, I learned to force myself to take a ten minute break and lie down. This is a part of the healing process. I had to learn to back off on some things and let go of others entirely. The main thing was to start somewhere. One baby step at a time.

Being a perfectionist, the demands I made on myself weren't even realistic and sometimes they weren't even rational. I had convinced myself my life was going to go better if I had done all those things. Somehow I thought I'd be a better person or I'd be happier. I couldn't win at this game.

Even though I'd been working fifteen hours a day, someone might say, "That's better, but it's still not quite good enough." When I managed a beauty school, the corporation I worked for made me quite frustrated. They always wanted a higher bottom line. I had to learn to set limits for myself.

Most workers are left with the task of deciding what is a reasonable day's work? Being a perfectionist at all levels, some people work themselves to death, to the point their supervisors have to say, "You've got to start going home at night. You're a wreck."

Being a perfectionist is such an internal thing that it's very hard for me to change. Even though I talk about it and joke about it and am working on it, I still have a hard time changing my ways. Somewhere, down deep inside, I was convinced that unless I kept doing things a certain way, that something bad was going to happen. Unfortunately, what happens with a lot of perfectionistic people is they burn out. They are very unhappy and depressed. They may have a very productive work history which will usually go in fits and starts. They start something looking like a shining star, and then may crash or fail miserably when they can't maintain the level of performance they expect of themselves or others.

Unfortunately, what they tell themselves is they are not perfectionistic enough. So their solution to the problem becomes the problem. This is why perfectionism is dangerous. If this was my excuse for not doing better, then I had to think maybe what it was creating was my lack of efficiency. If I aimed for excellence and got good at it, like the athlete, I could become much more happy and productive.

Any employer knows if they have a calm, relaxed, undepressed happy work staff, they will be most productive. They can even let them goof off a little bit; let them take an extra break or longer lunch hour. If the employer treats them better, then they gain their respect and they will work a lot harder for them in the long run.

To break the perfectionism habit, I needed to plan and structure my time, including time to rest and relax. It seemed odd at first. It seemed like I was letting myself, my family, and everyone else down. I felt guilty and bad, all those yucky feelings that go with it. The internal things I believed were much more powerful than the people in my life.

As I began to change from being a perfectionist to accepting excellence instead, I oftentimes lost some friends along the way. They were people who were also perfectionists, but who still lived in that world of expecting others to be as perfect as they were. I had to learn to set new boundaries with them. I had to know when I had to quit doing something in order to be healthy for me, and sometimes they didn't understand why I couldn't be as perfect as they. For example, if they stayed and worked late and I went home, it sometimes caused a rift between us.   Perfectionists are a hard bunch to live with. It was hard, but some of those friends I simply had to let go of in order to take care of my own health.

All people in relationships have expectations for those relationships. There is nothing wrong with that. What I needed to decide for myself was whether those expectations of others were realistic for me. Obviously in an employment situation, if I didn't meet their expectations, I could be without a job. However, that might not have been the worst thing that could happen. I had to remember my health should always come first. Without that, where would I be?

However in an interpersonal situation, I could be without a mate or some significant other if my issues dominated our situation in a negative way. When I got right down to it, the decisions I made needed to be made for me, by me. There was no way to escape. It's my life I'm living, whether I like it or not. I can't please everyone. I can do it for a while, but sooner or later it would turn into crap.

I almost had to step out of what was my culturally ingrained way of looking at the world. As Americans, our basic point of view is, 'bigger and faster are better.' In other cultures, this isn't true. Our current society doesn't put much value in things like happiness and contentment. Yet we seem to put great stock in achieving and producing, where happiness and contentment supposedly lie.

I had to learn that no matter what people told me, no matter how important they told me it was, or how critical, or what kind of a bad person I was going to be if I didn't do it, I had to remember that I had to do what was right for me and my health, first and foremost.

It's important for perfectionists to examine what you can personally tolerate. Some people can tolerate a great deal. Some perfectionists are fine doing tremendous amounts of work. They aren't stressed out, angry, or anxious. They can deal with being a perfectionist. They aren't going overboard. However, if it is getting in the way, then it's a problem.

I was under pressure, and I was feeling stress about this stuff so I needed to look further back. In this quote, "Only the mediocre are always at their best," I could become mediocre so that I would be doing well. It all depends on what I can tolerate. I can enjoy life. I can have a good time by taking the time to smell the roses, instead of rushing from this to that. I made this a personal goal; to take time to enjoy each moment of each day. I shifted the goal from getting it done to having to do it, to simply enjoying it, whether it was being with my kids or something else.

I watched people with their kids and sometimes could tell it was a job they were forced to do by the way they acted. Some parents complain about all the stuff they have to do with their kids, even though it is voluntary that they became a parent. This is a fact of life.

Do you know what changed my life as I was driving my kids all over the place, to after school events, dances, and to play in billiard tournaments? For some time, I was ticked off about it, then I finally realized, this is my life. Those are my children, whom I love dearly. I wanted to be involved in what they were doing. I might as well enjoy them. They will be gone before I realize what has happened. I discovered I wanted to enjoy the time I had left with them before they went off to college.

The change wasn't necessarily in the task or the demand, but in my approach to what I was doing. Almost anything I did, I needed to approach as if I wanted to enjoy what I was doing. And interestingly enough, I found out I really did enjoy what I was doing.

I already knew happy workers were more productive. They were satisfied and felt like they were respected and that what they did had some meaning. They weren't pressured and didn't have anyone breathing down their neck to force them to get the job done. It took society a long time to figure that out.

Not being self-confident had a lot to do with me trying to be a perfectionist. It was sort of like the chicken and the egg. Most of these things are circular. Being self-confident is the belief I can do something. It's a belief in myself. I needed to get in touch with myself. If I was constantly demanding the impossible of myself, and constantly setting myself up for failure, then eventually I would have no self-confidence. I needed to work on striving to achieve excellence in place of trying to be perfect. When I do this, my self-confidence goes up. I feel much better about myself and happier with my loved ones as I became a happier person in general. I have found out I can't make anybody else happy unless I'm happy with myself.

CATHERINE'S SUCCESS STORY

Treating Complex Regional Pain Syndrome

"The pain was so bad I took six to eight narcotic pain tablets a day. They didn't relieve the pain and I was 'out of it,' but I kept taking them because it was the only thing I could do. After receiving an Advanced Pain Therapy (APT) Neurostimulation, I experienced 60% relief on my breakthrough pain. Now I can sleep at least four hours at a time, and I only need pain medication and anti-inflammatory medication occasionally."

Catherine, a forty-four year old registered nurse injured her left shoulder while at work. She later developed reflex sympathetic dystrophy, RSD, also called Complex Regional Pain Syndrome or CRPS. Catherine initially received many treatments including nerve blocks, physical therapy, and a series of prescription drugs. But none of these therapies relieved her pain.

Because Catherine had pain in her arm, her doctors felt she was a good candidate for APT Neurostimulation. Catherine underwent a screening test, in which the doctor placed a lead, a special medical wire, at the level of her spine that corresponded to where she felt pain. She experienced sixty percent pain relief. The doctor then placed a permanent system two weeks later.

Since receiving the system, Catherine has continued to experience 60% pain relief. Some pain remains, and she takes an occasional pain reliever, where she had previously been taking six to eight pain relieving tablets per day. Although she still suffers for RSD, APT Neurostimulation has helped Catherine sleep better, and she is able to be more active. She is involved in occupational retraining so she can perform other nursing functions and plans to return to work.

Will I be able to adjust my Neurostimulation system?

The totally implantable system has a patient programmer, (similar to a computer mouse), that allows you to adjust the stimulation produced by the Neurostimulation system. In the radio frequency system, a transmitter similar to a pager allows you to adjust the system. This transmitter, with an antenna, needs to be worn at all times for the system to work.

The following may affect the function of your Neurostimulation system:

* magnetic resonance imaging (MRI)
* cardiac pacemakers
* therapeutic X-rays
* ultrasound
* defibrillator
* diathermy
* radiation therapy
* lithotripsy

Always tell any medical personnel that you have an implanted Neurostimulation system.

CHAPTER FIFTEEN

Guit and Chronic Pain

"Then, when you failed in everything, when what you had slowly built up was blown away in a moment, and you must toilsomely begin again from the beginning; when your arm was weak, your step wavering, then you still held fast to you expectation of faith, which is victory."   *- Soren Kierkegaard*

Guilt is a series of thought processes that leave me feeling bad about myself. Believe it or not, we all manufacture our own guilt and we have no one to blame but ourselves. No one can make us feel guilt, or any other emotion for that matter. It is our perception of an incident or act which leads us to falling upon old thought patterns we have generally maintained for years, which leads us to the development of all emotional responses and feelings. Realizing that we are the only ones responsible for our feeling is sometimes frightening. Yet by the same token, understanding that we are not responsible for how others feel, can be quite freeing at the same time.

It would be a very frightening world if I was responsible for how anyone else felt. That would be depressing. My feelings were due to lots and lots of things besides what I said or did or didn't do, including changing my mind. As I said before, "It is all a matter of opinion." There is no right or wrong. Most of us have ethical or moral beliefs. I do believe there is a right or wrong, although it isn't necessarily facts.

I could get extreme, like the Ten Commandments. "Thou shall not kill." Most everyone knows or has heard of someone who has killed another human being.

"Well, that's what happened in the war in Vietnam." What happened to that commandment? Some would say there were exceptions to that commandment.

People said "I would never kill anybody."

Imagine if you heard a noise in your house and you happened to have a gun handy. You walked into your daughter's bedroom and there was this crazed person standing next to her bed and he was leveling a revolver at her head. What would you do? Most people, even passive people, wouldn't hesitate and would blow this monster away. The point is not that you want to shoot people, but that whatever you thought was right or wrong is open to judgment and opinion.

A lot of people think someone else is causing them to have guilt. For instance, if a person said something to me like, "You shouldn't have done that. That's wrong. What a moron, nobody does it that way. Why don't you do it the right way?" I could believe the other person saying these things is what caused me guilt. I thought they made me feel guilty. Depending on what I told myself, that was what maintained the guilt.

If I changed my thinking, the way I felt about the guilt could change. I would be in control of how I felt. Whether it was my husband, children, or friends, someone would always be telling me something. I can't stop people in my life from telling me I did things wrong or I didn't do it right, even a minor thing like leaving my glasses on the coffee table.

I needed to look at the thinking part of the event. The guilt was coming from there. Most of my concerns were interpersonal. When I got right down to it, it was about relationships which are very often complicated from a judgment point of view.

That's the thing about guilt; once I started taking responsibility for my own guilt, then I was in charge. No one could make me feel guilt. I could be relatively un-guilty surrounded by people working day and night to make me feel guilty. That may be their sole job in life, to make me miserable for what ever reason. A lot of people are good at that stuff, but now, I know the secret. It doesn't work on me anymore, since I know I'm responsible for my own guilt.

Guilt is a control thing. Most parents are good at it. I am an adult, making my own money, raising my own children, and I have these parents who still give me a difficult time with a simple phone call. "So when are you going to come and visit us?"

"It's a very busy time, I'm really busy with the kids and our business."

"You hardly ever come and visit us. You know a daughter should visit her mom, especially when she's getting up in years."

This would go on and on and on until I was racked with guilt.

I talked to my friends and many of them had the same problem. They gave me advice. "Well, go visit them, call her more often."

Then other people said, "Forget it, you've tried."

So I get this whole spectrum. I wasn't saying any of these were right or wrong. But I couldn't settle it by going around and asking other people. Everybody would tell me something different. What did it all mean? It meant we all have different opinions. Some of them are helpful and some are totally useless.

So did I think it was possible or impossible to reduce my level of guilt? It is quite possible. I had to slow down, because I would automatically think a certain way. It depended on how I had been taught about a lot of things. This could "*increase*" my pain sometimes, but if I used it in the best way for me, it could also "*decrease*" my chronic pain.

There is no doubt in my mind that if I can reduce the feeling of guilt by how I think, then I can reduce the intensity of my chronic pain. I am responsible for all my feelings and shouldn't spend a lot of time worrying about what other people think. There are certain people who are extremely important to me. I care about what they think. I listen and seek out their information and advice, but others I could care less about what they think.

Guilt is a part of self-blame. For instance, if it wasn't for my chronic pain, I could be out working on location and having fun playing pool and living my life like I used to. I was labeling the guilt as my chronic pain, only causing myself more pain by the way I thought about my condition. People were always telling me how I should be living my life. Sometimes the best thing I could do was to go off by myself and do nothing until I had time to think things through and began to believe in myself.

At times, my family knew how to get me to feel guilty. They tended to make me feel it was my fault I had chronic pain and it was my fault I couldn't work anymore. Of course I loved my family and would do anything for them. Many of us feel this way.

The interpersonal relationships are the toughest. I had to be able to say, "No!" and mean it. My family turned away from me for a while, but they came back after they had time to think about what I was trying to do with my life.

It takes time for people who don't have pain to understand what a person with chronic pain has to deal with. The challenge was me telling them and standing up for myself.

An example would be when someone would say, "I have to have this done now." They could get very demanding. The question was why did they have to have it done now? They'd look at me and say, "Because it's important."

"I realize it's important, but why do you have to have it done right now?"

"Well, I want to have it done."

"Want is a different matter."

If I could get the person to be more clear about what they really were talking about, then I had a chance of getting out of it, especially with family members. I needed to hold people to what they meant. I said to people, "What do you mean I should do this?"

"It would be a good idea if you did it."

"I agree with you, it would be a good idea if I did it, but I choose not to do it."

"Well, you should do it."

"I lost you, what do you mean?"

"Well, it would be the right thing to do."

"You mean you *think* it would be the right thing to do."
"Obviously, I don't, or I'd be doing it."

"So, anybody knows it would be the right thing to do."

A lot of people used the looseness of their thinking and how they used words to get me. If I wanted to knock those words out of other people's vocabulary I would kindly say, "I don't understand. It's mysterious to me when I really think about it. You tell me I should do this. I would like to know by what authority? Is this constructive criticism? Would you like to reword this so I don't get upset? Were you telling me something you think I should consider? It sounded like you were giving me a command." After this the person usually reconsiders and becomes rational about what I'm doing.

Chronic pain is a limit setting, lifelong experience. Where ever I want to set my limits, it's okay. I'm not advocating being this tough, 'I don't care' type of person, because that isn't what I value personally. What I'm saying is I need to look inside myself to see what I am willing to tolerate, and find out what my limits are. I will be setting those limits for myself. I taught the people in my life how to treat me by how I would let them treat me. People couldn't treat me in a certain way if I didn't allow them to treat me that way. It's a hard lesson to learn, because it's much more comfortable to believe there wasn't anything I could do about it.

I had to watch when I started setting limits that I didn't let anger creep into my thoughts. I could remain kind and compassionate when I left out the anger. It's an old pattern and I wasn't able to do it without some real rough spots. At times, I wondered how I could change myself at this phase of the game. It all depended on whether I thought I could change. If I didn't think I could change, then I might as well give up trying, because it wouldn't work. If I thought I could change, (and I believed anybody could change anything if they wanted to change bad enough), then I could do it.

It was like anything else I was working on to get better. It needed to be a concerted day to day effort that I kept track of on a constant basis. I needed to work on it, because it wouldn't happen overnight.

Good things take time and time is something I had an abundance of. The first change in attitude I had to make was to accept that I was responsible for my own guilt. So if I had a high level of guilt, I'd better start doing something about it right then and there. I wouldn't waste as much of my time going around finding who I should blame for my guilt. Once I didn't respond in the way that was expected, by my family, they would about lose their minds. When I said, "Are you trying to get me to do this?" They said, "Oh, no," but they expected me to do what they wanted anyway. I read somewhere guilt is the iron fist inside a velvet glove. This is so true, especially with family members.

Journal Entry, June 16, 1996
Worst day I've had in a long time. Rob is depressed and I'm depressed. It was such a crazy day. He got mad at me because I wasn't playing Monopoly good enough with the kids. A really dumb thing. I know he's uptight about taxes, trying to get new financing on one of the buildings, and the business itself, since I haven't been able to work.

For a short time, I felt guilty about the whole thing. He thought I was going crazy and I wasn't. I was going through learning how to live with chronic pain.

I don't know if we're going to make it, if he really feels this way. He talks like I've ruined his life when I'm the one with the pain that affects us all.

Either it will work out or it won't. I'm not going to feel guilty about this disagreement when I know I'm doing the best I can do. I refuse to make my pain intensify because of something so silly.

Once I took responsibility for my guilt, and started looking out for myself, my life changed. I learned to set some limits and lived by them and told my family so. They were people I dearly loved, but I wasn't willing or able to do certain things anymore, and if that would be the end of the relationship, then that was the end. I had to remember I was fighting for my life. I didn't want our relationship to end, but if they couldn't accept my limits then I wouldn't be able to function in the relationship.

I'm not talking about a rational process. I'm talking about people trying to get other people to do things they want them to do. It isn't because they are mean or insensitive. They are only in the habit of using that style to get their way or control others. It has happened to a lot of us. I can't argue with the effectiveness of this style. However, it can have some pretty horrible side effects. We could have ended up hating each other. At one point I wanted to strangle all of them. Then I finally decided I didn't care any more. Then I was free.

I had to pay attention and the next time I felt guilty, I would check my head and see what I was telling myself. It was hard, but I did relearn ways of doing things. Guilt is a negative way of getting things done. I had to get the demand words *'should not,'* *'must,'* *'have to,'* and *'need to,'* out of my life. The less guilt I felt, the better I felt physically. Positive reward generates more reward. This all helped me to feel better.

CHAPTER SIXTEEN

Acceptance of the Devil's Curse

"These things I have spoken to you, that in Me you may have peace. In the world you have tribulation, but take courage; I have overcome the world." - *John 16:33 Be the rule and guide of your life in Jesus Christ. Amen*

To me, chronic pain is the Devil's curse. It is my personal curse which I am destined to live with for the rest of my days. Because life won't wait, I have accepted it and I have learned to deal with it. Life went on around me, passing me by until I was in control of myself and my life. I was put here to share my experience with others who have to live with pain daily. Believe me, it can be managed! I will never be the person I was physically, but perhaps I have become a better person for the understanding I now have and the appreciation of the world around me.

As I have grown through knowledge, I have found the positive side of life. It would have been easy to turn into a mean, bitter person blaming the world for my fate. In my heart, I know sometimes unpleasant things happen. There is no one else to blame. This came with the acceptance of my situation which brought me peace. Once I accepted my fate, I began to change. This was the first major step I had to take.

By writing this book I have taken another step. The writing has been a form of therapy for me. I didn't want to forget all the good things I had been taught and found it amazing what the human spirit can overcome if the person is shown the way. I am on my way to healing. Many people with chronic pain have died before their time. I know it isn't my time yet. I have too much life left in me to let the pain win. As in many things in life, it takes courage to accept and grow through perseverance. I have found chronic pain to be a journey, not a destination. When I graduated from the Pikes Peak Pain Program I knew what I was capable of doing and what I needed. I knew what I could do and what I couldn't do.

My family had to trust my judgment as an adult, with my own grown up decisions to make about how I was going to live my life. They couldn't do it for me and I couldn't do it for them. If they made all my decisions for me then my independence would have been limited. It could have gotten to the point where I would have been totally dependent on them. That would've killed me.

They had to listen to me about my frustrations, anxieties, plans, or questions the pain had caused me. Sometimes, when they shut up and listened, they learned a lot. This doesn't mean only families, but if my friends listened to what I was saying, they could learn a lot, too. Most of us have a tendency to talk and not really take the time to hear the other person, because we like to talk about ourselves and our own situations.

I really needed to listen to the other people in my family and they needed to listen to me. After I went through the pain program, plans were being made for my future. It was important to pay attention to those things. I needed to be real clear and open as to what my plans were all about to my family and friends.

For instance, if someone with chronic pain is planning to drive across the country and their family isn't sure they can handle the drive, it isn't realistic to let the person go ahead with those plans. A family member needs to speak up and say, "I think we need to talk about this a little more." With the help of my family, I had to rethink my plans many times before I was sure of what I could do.

In reality, nobody knows what is going to happen today, tomorrow, or next week. For those of us with chronic pain, it is harder to make plans. When I don't know what my physiological state of body is going to be, or what my emotional state of mind will be, it becomes an individual challenge.

One of the main goals of my family is acceptance. Acceptance of the fact this pain is going to stay around. This is a fact. This is where I'm at. The pain isn't going anywhere. It's here to stay for the rest of my life.

Once my family and I accepted this as a fact, I could go on. Acceptance was the single most important factor in moving ahead. Accepting this was where I was at in my life. I wasn't saying things couldn't change. I had been encouraged by the people with the Pikes Peak Pain Program to keep trying, keep doing, keep stretching, keep striving and to extend my limits a little bit farther each day. I was pleasantly surprised at what I could accomplish when I put my mind to it. In fact, the basic problem wasn't going to go away. So once my family and I accepted the fact I'd have this problem for the rest of my life, then and only then, the battle was beginning to be won.

Dealing with expectations is hard for everybody and being honest with myself and the people I cared about was real important. I had to make my expectations something I could do. I had to be fair with myself and my family.

One patient in the pain program wanted to jog for her exercise. To go back to running would be hard. That wasn't saying the person would never run again. She might jog or do better than she was doing at the time. However, running wasn't a realistic expectation. It was a fun idea, but it probably wasn't going to work, but who knows, maybe she could do it. The mind is a powerful thing.

Accepting the challenge that I had challenges, and being realistic about what I could do gave me a chance to improve things. I am improving on a daily basis.

I had to think of chronic pain as an opportunity to grow. I had learned things I always knew. They were always there at the back of my mind. Just as I had always known I needed to communicate better with everyone. I learned to think of this as an opportunity. This was a chance to put forth things I'd always known, but didn't take the time to put them into action.

I had always thought about improving my relationship with my husband and children and working on my communications with everyone. Sometimes this became too much work and I let these things go. After better understanding chronic pain, I picked myself up and started over.

Thinking of this as an opportunity for things to improve with my family, we have become closer through these trials and difficulties. Any family can become closer if they work on it together. We found faith and strength in each other.

I was off all the drugs, and increasing my awareness on a day-to-day basis. I saw and felt the changes happening to me and learned what I could do in a positive way to sustain those changes and to help me make new changes. My awareness emotionally, physically, and psychologically increased on a daily basis. Being aware of my own feelings and the feelings of the people I was most involved with was very important. Developing understanding was something we could work on together. It seemed to help when we thought of this as having an opportunity to be more understanding with each other.

Before I reacted, I had to think about the situation for a second and examine my capabilities to understand what was really going on, and maybe by doing this, I could make things a little bit more successful. We all had to try and understand each other more. My husband and children couldn't possibly put themselves in my shoes but they could make efforts to understand me. The survival of my family absolutely, positively, was improving.

A lot of families don't like improvement. They tend to resist change. This isn't an easy task. This stuff isn't something that happens magically. They aren't going to walk out and wave everything suddenly okay. It takes a lot of work. Families have to learn how to talk about things without getting angry.

When I came in to be evaluated for the Pikes Peak Pain Program I was told by everyone there wasn't a cure for chronic pain. Yet, when other patients, including myself, started the program, they still chose to think there was. People don't hear what they don't want to hear. A lot of time people don't even ask the question of whether it is curable or not. They choose to ignore the whole thing. This is their mind set. Without recognizing what the problem is and knowing what I could do about it, I couldn't fix the problem. A fix was not in the future, but magic was. I could live with that on a day to day basis. At the time, it didn't matter how real it was.

I learned how to listen so I could hear what was really being said to me. Sometimes when someone was talking I used to try and think ahead of this person and have a response ready for them before they were through speaking. Most of us are guilty of doing this at some time. I had to slow down and listen. I might have had to ask questions to find out if what I heard was what was meant for me to hear, and what was really the understanding of the way it was. A lot of times it wasn't the same thing.

It was very hard for my family to not do things for me, even if it was for my own good. Other times it was better for them to say, "Can I help you do that?" This way I could at least put forth some effort to try to improve, but not have to do it all. They had to try to think of this as assessing their judgment. They tried to show me they had the confidence in me to let me try to do things.

With practice, everybody who has chronic pain can manage their life on their own without any help from anybody.

There is a big shift for the family when the person with chronic pain graduates from the program and goes home and starts doing things for themselves, again. It is a learning experience for everyone involved. Families have to make some changes in the way they've been treating each other.

My suggestion for the families would be to trust that your loved one with chronic pain can do it, whatever it might be. They are capable of doing things for themselves. The family members have to trust their loved one's judgment. Let them do what they want to do. Unless they ask you for help, don't give it. Have enough confidence in them to believe they can manage themselves. Allow them to do the same for you. Treat them as responsible adults. Family members have to believe the chronic pain person can take care of themselves.

A lot of times, families start out being loving and caring, yet when the illness continues on for a year or two, they decide this is getting old. They are tired and the person with chronic pain is less and less help, and less and less co-operative. Not only did they not get help, but they were sometimes ignored. The chronic pain patient even starts to feel mistreated and may even do things to see if their loved ones come to help them.

Then when their loved ones came to help they said, "Get out of here, I want to do things for myself." This is sending mixed signals to the family. Their pain behavior is showing they need help, yet they are in denial they need the help.

The person with chronic pain doesn't want to admit they are disabled. This is an example of a double bias. Your loved one is in a no-win situation. They are so confused with your signals they don't know what to do to help you.

The person with chronic pain has to allow themselves to take responsibility for the healing process. I had to be more honest with myself and my family. Otherwise, nobody knew what to do. In the early stages of chronic pain, I didn't understand when it was okay to ask for help. What I was doing wasn't meant to be mean or hateful or deceitful. I got into a condition where I didn't know what to do and my family didn't know what I wanted from them. I didn't know who to ask for help. The frustration of the pain only made me more hurt and angry.

In the beginning, my loved ones didn't know how much help to give me. They didn't know how much pain I was in, or how much they could do for me. With what they learned with me at the pain program, they now know they can do some things, but before that, they didn't understand when it was okay to help and not okay to help. It was frustrating for everyone concerned.

This was where the trust came into the situation. After leaving the program, the person with chronic pain has learned his or her limits. They know when to ask for help so the families have to trust their judgment and let them ask for help when they need it.

The people who need help must ask and the people who are willing to offer help, should do so when asked, and not before. This way they don't have to assume they know when the family member needs help and it's much easier on everyone concerned.

Thanks to the Pikes Peak Pain Program, I learned what I needed to survive. My family and I were able to continue our healing process together. Because of what all of us had gone through learning to live with chronic pain we are closer than we ever were.

At my graduation from the pain program my husband made the following comment:

"At this time I would like to thank everybody involved for giving me my wife back. I'm sure my kids feel the same way. We always knew she could make it back and I know it has taken a lot of everybody's time and effort.

"I remember going through basic training and being in a situation like this where it was real stressful and I deeply relied on everybody around me to pull me through. If I didn't have people then I would've gone off on a tangent. I wanted to run away and hide. I couldn't do it. I knew I couldn't do it. This was all I could tell myself. It wasn't going to happen. Then the guy next to me said, 'You can do it, if I can do it, you can do it.' It snowballed and before I knew it, I was through it. "I fall back on those times so many instances in my life that it's amazing.

"I think about those times a lot when I have something hard to do. I know that this is similar to what she's going through and she wouldn't be where she's at now without everybody in the Pikes Peak Pain Program doing for each other. I appreciate everything you've all done for my wife, I really do."

A comment from my fourteen year old son, Robert J. Willhoff III: *"It's great to have my mom back. Thanks for helping her."*

A comment from my thirteen year old daughter, Jennifer Willhoff: *"I'd like to say I'm glad my mom found this program. Before, she'd sit in her recliner all day in pain and be grouchy and stuff. It's true. I can definitely see a change in my mom. She's happy, again, which has made us all happy."*

To me, those comments from my family said it all. I didn't realize what was happening to me when it all began. I had been trapped in a never ending nightmare. Now, I have control of my life. I still have chronic pain, but I am in charge of my condition. I have learned how to deal with it in the right way.

Instead of ending my life, with God on my side, I chose to fight back. During my journey, I discovered more than eighty-six million people have been diagnosed with chronic pain. That's one out of three. Many who weren't fortunate enough to find help have committed suicide, as I could have easily done.

I have learned to take nothing for granted in life, because it can all be taken away in an instant. I take the time to appreciate the little joys...going for a walk in the warm sunshine...smelling a rose, or holding my newborn grandchild. It's truly amazing what the human spirit can do with the help of God. In adversity, I was able to renew my faith and strengthen my bond with God.

Thanks to my prayers being answered, I have a new heart of love, hope, and strength. I have a new purpose for myself with a higher quality of existence I didn't have before this experience. I have been to the edge of suicide and survived. If I can do it, you can, too.

SAM'S SUCCESS STORY

Treating Pain Due to Arachnoiditis

Pain had become a part of everyday life for Sam. It started when he cracked three vertebrae in his neck during a parachute jump in Vietnam—and nearly ended when worn out from incessant pain, Sam attempted to take his own life.

"I thought it was the only way I could get through the pain," Sam said. Luckily, a friend was able to help him seek medical care.

Sam has Arachnoiditis, an inflammation of the membrane covering the spinal cord that causes severe pain by pressing on the nerves. After years of pain medication and failed surgeries, an anesthesiologist specializing in pain management proposed they try Medtronic Advanced Pain Therapy Intrathecal.

Two weeks after a successful screening test, Sam underwent surgery to begin Advanced Pain Therapy Intrathecal. He experienced no complications, and went home the day following the procedure.

"Now my wife and I can go out to dinner when we want," Sam said. "We go out with friends, go to football games and baseball games—different things that I haven't been able to do in years." Sam is also able to help in his family's business.

Sam has experienced no side effects from the therapy. He credits Advanced Pain Therapy Intrathecal with helping him escape from a life of debilitating pain.

"This pump is really helping me. I have some bad days, but most are good days. It's nice to have the chance to enjoy my life again."

Will Medtronic Advanced Pain Intrathecal completely eliminate my pain?

While it may not be possible to completely eliminate your pain, APT Intrathecal may help you control it so you are more comfortable. Your doctor may prescribe additional oral medication to relieve pain which occasionally "breaks through" the treatment.

CHAPTER SEVENTEEN

Choosing a Pain Management Doctor

**"Some days are diamonds...some days are rocks
Some doors are open...some roads are blocked."
- *Tom Petty***

Checking out a pain management doctor's credentials is very important. I had to be assertive in a nonaggressive manner. Finding a doctor to treat chronic pain can be very frustrating. With my health insurance policy, they tend to try to limit choices. Many insurance companies spend a lot of time trying to avoid their obligations. They are great until you become ill and need them.

I asked my family physician for assistance in choosing a pain management doctor I could feel most comfortable with. Always remember, there are choices. A patient should always explore their options for treatment. I had to ensure the chosen doctor was qualified to practice the treatment I needed or wanted.

In my search for a good chronic pain doctor I interviewed several. I talked to them and saw whether they were the kind of doctor I wanted to have.

Taking the time to check out the doctor's credentials was important to me. I had to make sure they were board certified in pain management. I had to be assertive. After all, this was my life. Finding a pain doctor I could trust took time.

By this time, I knew what was wrong with my body and knew what I needed. I was only making sure I got adequate care. I would have to monitor myself so I didn't go overboard on medication or treatment. I had to make sure I had a qualified doctor taking care of me.

If I was in the waiting room or treatment room and it just didn't look clean, then I'd know this wasn't where I wanted to be. There are always indicators as to what type of doctor I was dealing with.

I don't think physical medicine is the only type of medicine there is on this earth. There are all kinds of doctors. To name a few, there are faith healers, people who lay hands on, people who use herbs to cure certain things, hypnotists, and many others. Maybe some of these could work for me, but I believe in traditional medicine. The main thing to remember, no matter what kind of doctor I believe in, was it was my responsibility to check that person out. I had to be sure I was seeing a qualified doctor with credentials. I couldn't afford to get stuck with someone who would take me for an expensive ride.

When the time came for my consultation, I looked for a doctor who listened to me, and told me his recommendations. Then I decided if he was a doctor I felt comfortable taking care of me. I had to remember these doctors were human, too. They weren't God. I'd learned they all can make mistakes.

Because of the friendship with my family physician, Dr. Higgins, I was lucky. He looked out for me. He was like my home base I would always return to. I had been his patient for over ten years and I trusted him. When all my testing was completed and the diagnosis made, he knew when it was time to send me to a specialist, he didn't deal with my type of disease.

Any time I saw another doctor, I had them send back a report to Dr. Higgins so he could keep up with what was happening with my case. I knew I had someone there I could trust to let me know if I was getting off track. Having a personal physician I could trust, was one of the most important things to me as I was learning to deal with my chronic pain. Not only did he look out for my physical condition, but his office also made sure the specialist or whoever I saw was covered by my health insurance. All those tests and treatments are quite expensive. As an individual, I need all the help I can get when it comes to understanding insurance coverage.

When I went through the Pikes Peak Pain program, reports were sent to Dr. Higgins, my primary care doctor, and I chose Dr. Charles Ripp, one of the best in the field, as my pain management doctor.

The main thing to remember is to be aware and know you are the boss. It's your choice as to who you want to have as your chronic pain doctor. In some cases, even though the doctor I want might not be on my insurance list, the company might let me have him if he is a specialist I need for my condition.

I would never be able to do the job I did before chronic pain. This was another lifestyle change I had become accustomed to. When I left the pain program I was at (MMI), Maximum Medical Improvement. What this meant, at that point in time, was that the physician felt I'd gotten the best results I was going to get. This was all he could do for me.

After the doctors had diagnosed and treated me and they felt I was at a level where there was no more possible improvement, I went through an evaluation process. The doctor recommended a Function Capacity Evaluation, (FCE). Results of this test determined my impairment rating. After FCE results, I was given a (MMI) Maximum Medical Improvement Rating. This rating was determined based on my percentage of disability.

I was considered 100% disabled and didn't have any idea of what I'd do after I left the clinic. I tried not to dwell on that and put my health first. That would all come in good time. My health came first.

I was thankful to have a family physician I could trust. He would always be there to get me back on track health wise when the road got rough. Thank God for Dr. Higgins and his staff and their support during my journey.

As far as my career, it was a thing of the past. I used to work as a freelance make-up artist, doing hair, make-up, wardrobe, and special effects for movies and commercials. When I wasn't doing that, I worked in our real estate office. Now, after going through the pain treatment center I am able to work in our real estate business part time and pursue other interests. I trust in God to show me another way. Where there's a will, there's a way. When one door closes, another will open. I keep my faith and take things one day at a time.

CHAPTER EIGHTEEN

Chronic Pain Syndrome: What is it?

"Above all, do not lose your desire to walk: every day I walk myself into a state of well being and walk away from every illness. I walked myself into my best thoughts so burdensome that one cannot walk away from it....The more one sits still, the closer one comes to feeling ill....Thus if one keeps on walking, everything will be all right." -*Soren Kierkegaard (Letter to Jette - 1847)*

Even though there is no cure for Chronic Pain Syndrome, it can be managed. With proper support and learning lifestyle changes, patients can come to rely on themselves and live a full rewarding life. I didn't know how to react when I was told I had Chronic Pain Syndrome. It didn't get any easier; there were always obstacles to overcome. There are more than eighty-six million people who have chronic pain. With the Baby Boomer generation getting older, there are more injuries and cases of this being diagnosed everyday. It comes down to one out of three people having this condition. I wasn't alone.

Dr. Kevin C. Murphy Ph.D., the Clinical Director of the Pikes Peak Pain Program has kindly consented to let me include here an article he has had published in the American Journal of Pain Management. I feel this article is invaluable to those who are physically experiencing Chronic Pain Syndrome and to those family members and loved ones who are struggling with the acceptance and understanding of this debilitating disability.

AJPM Vol. 4 No. 3 July 1994

COMMENTARY

CHRONIC PAIN SYNDROME: WHAT IS IT, AND HOW CAN WE HELP?
By Kevin C. Murphy, Ph.D.

Abstract. Chronic Pain Syndrome is a well-recognized problem. Many attempts to explain its development, evaluation, and subsequent management have been too simplistic. Any meaningful description of the problem must include an acknowledgment of the many interconnected, secondary issues associated with this syndrome. Successful interventions are best accomplished by an interdisciplinary team of experts that can capably evaluate and reduce the impact of the secondary problems on the individual's functioning. Until more widespread agreement is reached among the many professionals working with this seemingly treatment-resistant syndrome, pain management practitioners will not significantly reduce its impact on those afflicted.

Descriptors. Chronic pain syndrome, interdisciplinary, learned behavior, pain management
AJPM 1994;4:129-131. Received: 2-1-94; Accepted: 4-21-94

The scene is all too familiar. A troubled individual complains of constant, severe pain that interferes with activities in which the individual had previously been engaged. The pain has not been relieved by any attempts at amelioration to date, and any sustained movement only worsens the pain. Consequently, a thick file of inconclusive diagnostic tests and failed treatments has been amassed. The desperate search for a cure has extended for months, and the individual appears depressed, angry, and anxious about increasing loss, frustration, and uncertainty.

Such a challenge is variously labeled as chronic intractable benign pain (1), somatoform pain disorder (2), or more inclusively, Chronic Pain Syndrome (3). The condition of Chronic Pain Syndrome (CPS) is clearly recognized as a significant problem in its own right—a problem that is far more devastating than the injury that initiated it (4).

While many have attempted to make sense of this baffling and seemingly treatment-resistant problem, most descriptions have greatly simplified this complex condition. One recent attempt exhorts practitioners to differentiate three groups of persons with pain: those with physically-based pain, those with psychogenic pain, and those who do not have pain, but claim they do (5). In clinical practice, however, practitioners regularly see persons with all three of these factors— sometimes more—maintaining their pain and physical dysfunction. A more complete conceptualization of the problem needs to incorporate these and other interconnected, secondary difficulties that develop in the wake of continued pain following reasonable treatments.

As time passes, these additional problems multiply and become ingrained habits of behavior (6).

CPS is first distinguished by what it is not. It is imperative to realize that CPS shares next to nothing with the more familiar problem of acute pain. While the two often begin in the same manner (i.e., injury), the clear progression of acute pain from definitive diagnosis, through effective treatment, to cure clearly distinguishes it from chronic pain. Almost all treatments and procedures used to assist patients with acute pain are entirely inappropriate for patients with chronic pain. (Table 1). In most cases, approaching chronic pain as if it were acute actually exacerbates the situation. The attempted solution, then, sadly becomes part of the ongoing problem.

The central or core problems of CPS is the presence of persistent pain over time despite reasonable treatment. Predictably, learned secondary problems collect over this time span as a direct result of ongoing, intractable pain. These secondary problems (Figure 1) are physical, psychological, social, and vocational. They overlay and interact in a personal fashion to produce the enigmatic array of behaviors that describe Chronic Pain Syndrome. Inactivity, depression with its lack of initiation, family conflict, and disruption of work are common. While any single treatment modality may address one or two of these secondary problems, such discipline-specific interventions do not consider the directly related factors that may, in turn, be affected. For instance, prescribing a back brace may prevent the chronic pain sufferer from performing a favored activity (e.g., gardening), resulting in increased depression. The brace may also signal to loved ones that the person is "broken" and helpless. And, it may convince an employer that the person is unable to return to work.

Conceptualizing CPS as an interconnected collection of learned secondary problems acquired over time suggests an optimal evaluation procedure. It is necessary to assemble an interdisciplinary team with the expertise to access the scope and magnitude of all physical, psychological, social, and vocational problems maintaining the syndrome. The effectiveness of this interdisciplinary approach to the evaluation and subsequent treatment of chronic pain is well established (7).

Once the impact of the multitude of factors prolonging pain is described, appropriate treatment or management becomes clear. This must involve a team trained and experienced in the management of all the interrelated factors working cooperatively to systematically reduce their impact on the individual's pain and dysfunction. Such team members are not only experts in their own disciplines, but they all also agree on overall team and patient goals, and they work toward them cooperatively. The central goal for all involved is to diminish the negative effect of each secondary problem, thereby resulting in increased activity and endurance, improved mood, smoother family interactions, and the ability to sustain work.

It is imperative the pain management practitioners clearly and accurately describe the development, evaluation, and effective management of chronic pain syndrome. Without this first critical step, it is unlikely that clinicians will be able to reduce meaningfully the devastating effects of this costly problem.

TABLE 1.
DIFFERENCE BETWEEN ACUTE AND CHRONIC PAIN

ACUTE PAIN

1. Usually short in duration
2. Degree and intensity secondary to recent injury or disease
3. Single cause is typically evident
4. Rest and inactivity needed
5. Splinting useful
6. Pain medication helpful
7. Reliance on health care appropriate
8. Waiting for a cure is reasonable
9. Trying to find a cause is appropriate
10. Relief from responsibilities is reasonable

CHRONIC PAIN

1. Usually of extended duration
2. Degree and intensity secondary to time since injury
3. Multiple causes are typically evident
4. Rest and inactivity inappropriate
5. Splinting harmful
6. Pain medication potentially harmful
7. Reliance on oneself is appropriate
8. Understanding that no cure beyond working hard at change

is necessary

9. Realizing that causation is so complex that dwelling on it is a waste of time

10. Relief from responsibility leads to helplessness

FACTORS CONTRIBUTING TO CHRONIC PAIN

Factors/Persons Involved

1.PhysicalPhysician, Physical Therapist, Chiropractor, Dentist, Occupational Therapist

2. PsychologicalPsychologist, Psychiatrist, Marriage Counselor

3. SocialSocial Worker, Case Worker, Friend

4. Vocational Employer, Attorney, Worker's Compensation

COMPLEXITY OF CHRONIC PAIN

1. Reconditioning and marked inactivity
2. Pessimism and depression
3. Marital and family problems
4. Loss of role as a worker
5. Weight gain
6. Anger and hostility
7. Attention and support for being in pain
8. Getting paid for doing nothing
9. Tissue, muscle and nerve damage from injury
10. Fear and loss of control
11. Lack of recreation and social interaction
12. Complex legal issues related to compensation
13. Erratic sleep patterns
14. Passivity and dependence

15. Financial problems
16. Pressure from employer and insurance company
17. Dependence on pain medication
18. Distrust and suspiciousness

Kevin C. Murphy Ph.D. is the Clinical Director at the Pikes Peak Pain Program of Colorado Springs in Colorado.

REFERENCES

1.Crue BL, Pinsky JJ. An approach to chronic pain of non-malignant origin. Postgrad Med J 1984;60:858-864

2.American Psychiatric Association. Diagnostic and statistical manual of mental disorders III. Washington DC: American Psychiatric Association, 1987

3.Weintraub MI. Litigation - chronic pain syndrome - a distinct entity: analysis of 210 cases. AJPM 1992;2:198 - 204.

4.Melzack R, Wall P. The challenge of pain. New York: Basic Books, 1982.

5.Lowe JC. Litigation - chronic pain syndrome: Weintraub's unproven entity. AJPM 193;3:131 - 136.

6.Fordyce WE, Fowler R. Lehmann J. De Lateur B. Some implications of learning in problems of chronic pain. J. Chronic Dis 1968;21:179 - 190

7.Arnoff GM. Evans WO, Enders PL. A review of follow-up studies of multidisciplinary pain units. Pain 1983;16:1 - 12.

CHAPTER NINETEEN

When Life Depends on Medical Technology

"God, give us the grace to accept with serenity the things that cannot be changed; Courage to change the things that should be changed; And the wisdom to distinguish the one from the other."
- Reinhold Niebuhr

Medtronic is a world leader in medical technology, pioneering pain therapies which restore health, extend life, and alleviate pain.

What is Pain?
It is the brain, not the point of injury that registers the sensation of pain. When you feel pain, it is really a reaction to signals that are transmitted throughout your body. These signals are sent from the pain source, through the nerves in the spinal cord, to your brain, where you perceive them as pain.

This is important because it means that pain can be controlled by preventing the pain signals from reaching the brain. If the pain signals never reach the brain, you don't feel the pain.

Different Types of Pain

The origin of some pain is neuropathic, while other pain is nociceptive. This is important to know because different treatments will work better for each type of pain.

Neuropathic pain is pain that is caused by damage to nerve tissue. It is often felt as a burning or stabbing pain. One example of a neuropathic pain is a "pinched nerve." Advanced Pain Therapy Neurostimulation is commonly used for neuropathic pain.

Nociceptive pain means pain caused by an injury or disease outside the nervous system. It is often an on-going dull ache or pressure, rather than the sharper, trauma-like pain more characteristic of neuropathic pain. Examples of chronic nociceptive pain include pain from cancer or arthritis. Advanced Pain Therapy Intrathecal is commonly used for nociceptive pain.

Some people experience mixed pain, which is a combination of neuropathic and nociceptive pain.

Barriers To Seeking Pain Relief

Many people with chronic pain don't seek pain relief, or even tell their doctors about their pain. Most often, the reasons for keeping pain a secret are based on fears or myths:

* Fear of being labeled as a "bad patient."

You won't find relief if you don't talk with your doctor about the pain you feel.

* Fear that increased pain may mean the disease has worsened. Regardless of the state of your disease, the right treatment for pain may improve daily life for you and your family.

* Fear of addiction to drugs.

Research has shown people with chronic pain can relieve pain without addiction.

* Lack of awareness about pain therapy options. Be honest about how your pain feels and how it affects your life. Ask your doctor about the pain therapy options available to you. Often, if one therapy isn't effectively controlling your pain, another therapy can.

* Fear of being perceived as "weak."

Some believe that living stoically with pain is a sign of strength, while seeking help often is considered negative or weak. This perception prevents them seeking the best treatment with available therapies.

Don't let fears and misconceptions keep you from talking to your doctor and other members of your health care team about getting adequate pain relief. Help and relief are possible, but only if you discuss your symptoms with your doctor.

What Are Medtronic Advanced Pain Therapies?

Thousands of people with chronic pain or cancer don't get enough pain relief, have uncomfortable side effects, or experience complications from oral medications or repeated surgeries. Medtronic Advanced Pain Therapies provide additional options for those people.

Advanced Pain Therapies (APT) are proven, effective alternatives to back surgery, drugs, or other therapies. APT Intrathecal and APT Neurostimultation works directly on the spinal cord—the highway for pain signals—and is thought to work by interfering with pain signals before they reach the brain. APT Neurostimulation can also work to electrically stimulate a peripheral nerve in patients with severe intractable pain. They can offer good to excellent pain relief, and can improve an individual's ability to go about daily activities. Your doctor can do a screening test, which helps predict whether the therapy will relieve your pain. In addition, both therapies are non-destructive and reversible.

Advanced Pain Therapy Neurostimulatin, including both spinal cord stimulation and peripheral nerve stimulation, uses a small neurostimulation system that is surgically placed under the skin to send mild electrical impulses to the spinal cord. The electrical impulses are delivered through a lead, a special medical wire, that is also surgically placed. These electrical impulses block the signal of pain from reaching the brain. Peripheral nerve stimulation works in a similar way, but the lead is placed on the specific nerve that is causing pain rather than near the spinal cord.

Because APT Neurostimulation works in the area where pain signals travel, electrical impulses, which are felt as tingling, can be directed to cover the specific sites where you are feeling pain. APT Neurostimulation can give patients effective pain relief and can reduce or eliminate the need for repeat surgeries and the need for pain medications.

Advanced Pain Therapy Intrathecal uses a small pump that is surgically placed under the skin of the abdomen to deliver morphine directly to the intrathecal space, the fluid around the spinal cord. The medication is delivered through a small tube called a catheter that is also surgically placed.

The spinal cord is like a highway for pain signals on their way to the brain, where the feeling of pain is experienced by your body. Because the drug is delivered right to the spinal cord, where pain signals travel, pain can often be dramatically controlled with a tiny fraction of the dose that would be required with pills. This helps minimize side effects.

Is APT Neurostimulation new?

Neurostimulation is not new. It has helped thousands of patients worldwide since its beginnings in the early 1970's. Medtronic, the first company to provide neurostimulation systems, continues to apply new medical technology to refine the systems.

What does APT Neurostimulation feel like?

The sensation felt from neurostimulation varies from person to person, but most report a tingling sensation in the area of their pain. Ideally, stimulation will provide a pleasant tingling sensation in the areas where you usually feel pain. However, neurostimulation does not mask sharp pain from a new injury.

Is APT Neurostimulation safe?

Clinical research has shown that the tiny electrical pulses from the neurostimulation system do not damage the nervous system. Likewise, research has shown that the materials in the electrodes and other implanted components are safe.

Are there any side effects to APT Neurostimulation?

Neurostimulation is not addictive and has no apparent side effects. Unlike some drugs used to control pain, neurostimulation does not cause drowsiness, disorientation, or nausea. And, it treats only the area where there is pain rather than affecting the entire body.

Will APT Neurostimulation completely eliminate my pain?

APT Neurostimulation does not eliminate the source of pain, so the amount of pain reduction varies from person to person. Your screening test will help your doctor see if neurostimulation will work for you. Typically, people who find the therapy helpful experience fifty to seventy percent pain relief. Those people who do not experience adequate relief generally will not receive a system as part of their pain therapy.

Neurostimulation is just one part in your pain therapy plan. The therapy requires a strong patient commitment to effectively control pain. Learning to operate the neurostimulation equipment and participating in other therapies, such as physical therapy, help ensure success.

What are the possible complications associated with APT Neurostimulation?

Any pain treatment can cause side effects. However, complication risks with APT Neurostimulation are low. Please discuss this with your doctor. APT Neurostimulation does require surgery. As with any surgery, some risks exist. These risks include:

. infection
. bleeding, hemorrhage
. headache
. hardware difficulties
. spinal cord injury
. allergic reactions
. failure to relieve pain
. paralysis
. hematoma
. pain at implant site

Some general complications that may be experienced with the system include:
. no stimulation or intermittent stimulation
. stimulation in the wrong location
. loss of pain relieving effect
. allergic response to system

How can APT Neurostimulation help me in my day-to-day activities?

APT neurostimulation may relieve your pain, allowing you to increase activities:
. traveling
. resuming sexual activity
. working at your home or job
. recreation such as walking, hiking, gardening, or fishing
. sleeping

Will I feel the Neurostimulation system inside me, and will people notice?

The IPG, internal battery, or receiver does not make any noise. It may be felt as a small bulge under your skin. It does not normally show through your clothes. The device is about 2.25 inches, 6 cm wide, 2 inches, 5.2 cm high, and one-half inch, 1cm thick. It is usually implanted in the lower abdomen, where it is most comfortable and least visible. You can discuss placement with your doctor before surgery and decide the best location for the IPG or receiver. If your doctor recommends a radio frequency system the transmitter will be visible and is usually worn on the belt like a pager. In addition, an antenna must be placed on your skin for the system to work.

Will my insurance company pay for the APT Neurostimulation?

The systems are approved by Medicare and many insurance carriers will pay for the Neurostimulation system. However, as with many therapies, your doctor will have to get approval from your insurance company before you can receive Neurostimulation. Consult your doctor or insurance carrier for more specific information.

Where can I get more information about APT?

Call the Medtronic Helpline at (800) 664-5111, ext.855 to request a packet of information about APT Intrathecal and APT Neurostimulation or go to www.Medtronic.com.

Frequently Asked Questions from People Receiving APT Neurostimulation

Will I be able to adjust my Neurostimulation system?

The totally implantable system has a patient programmer, similar to a computer mouse, that allows you to adjust the stimulation produced by the Neurostimulation system. In the radio frequency system, a transmitter similar to a pager allows you to adjust the system. This transmitter, with an antenna, needs to be worn at all times for the system to work.

Will I experience any changes in sensation?

Because APT Neurostimulations is positional, some patients may feel more changes than others. However, in general the sensation of stimulation remains constant. Some people may feel changes in sensation with sudden abrupt movements or shifts in posture. For example, when laying down you may feel stronger sensation because the lead is closer to the nerves of the spinal cord than when standing. Changes in stimulation are more common during the first several weeks after surgery.

How long will my totally implantable Neurostimulation system last?

This time varies. The battery life of the implanted pulse generator, IPG, depends on how many hours a day the system is used, the intensity of the stimulation, and individual differences. The screening test process will help you and your doctor decide whether an internally powered or externally powered system is best for your battery requirements.

How will I know when the battery on my totally implantable Neurostimulation system needs to be replaced?

Your doctor will be able to tell you the state of the battery in the Neurostimulation system during regularly scheduled follow-up visits.

What happens when my battery needs to be replaced?

When it is time to have your battery replaced, your doctor, using a minor surgical procedure, will remove the device and replace it with a new one. If you are using a radio frequency system, you simply replace the 9-volt battery in the transmitter. This is typically done on an outpatient basis.

When should I call my doctor about my Neurostimulation system?

Consult your doctor when:

*   you experience additional, unusual pain
*   you notice unusual changes in the quality of your stimulation or when you experience no sensation
*   you are increasing stimulation more often than normal
*   when the stimulation pattern changes

Otherwise, visit your doctor according to your follow-up schedule. A typical follow-up schedule is once every six months, although equipment may initially require more frequent adjustments. Your doctor may want to see you more or less frequently, depending on your stimulation.

What safety precautions should I follow with APT Neurostimulation?

With the Neurostimulation system, you can safely use most common household appliances, including microwave ovens, televisions, am/fm radios, stereos, remote controls, and video games.

Can my system be affected by strong magnetic equipment?

Yes, the totally implantable system can be affected by magnets. Because of this you should avoid being close to:

*   theft detectors

* airport/security screening devices
* large stereo speakers with magnets
* electric arc welding equipment
* high-voltage power lines
* electric substations and power generators

Magnets can turn some systems ON or OFF, but will not change the programmed stimulation settings. The security guard at the airport will wand the passengers so they won't have to go through the screening devices.

Will theft control devices affect my APT Neurostimulation system?

Some patients have experienced problems such as jolting or shocking stimulation with theft control devices at stores and libraries. If you are entering an area with a theft control device, please take the following precautions:

1. Move cautiously to within a couple of feet of the theft control device.

2. Turn your amplitude to zero, then turn your Neurostimulator off.

3. If you do not feel an increase in stimulation, pass through the center of the vertical detection panels of the system without stopping.

4. If you feel a sudden increase in your stimulation as you approach the theft detector, do not pass through the detector until the detector is turned OFF.

Will my system set off the metal detectors at the airport?

It might. You will receive an ID card that you can present to security personnel for clearance if necessary.

What medical procedures and equipment should I avoid?

The following may affect the function of your Neurostimulation system:

* magnetic resonance imaging (MRI)
* cardiac pacemakers
* X-rays
* ultrasound

* defibrillator
* diathermy
* radiation therapy
* lithotripsy

Always tell any medical personnel that you have an implanted Neurostimulation system.

Are there any special instructions for patients receiving APT Neurostimulation?

Strictly follow your doctor's instructions about proper body positioning, lifting, twisting, bending, stretching, and other activity to minimize problems. It is recommended you avoid extreme stretching or twisting the first six to eight weeks following your implant procedure. This allows the lead to become anchored in place. It is also important to keep all follow-up appointments as scheduled.

CHAPTER TWENTY

Frequently Asked Questions About
Advanced Pain Therapies

"What I don't know I will no longer allow to intimidate me. I will instead view it as an opportunity. I refuse to be shackled by yesterday's failures." - *Unknown*

How will my doctor know if I am a candidate for Advanced Pain Therapy?

Your doctor can do a screening test to help predict whether APT will relieve your pain. Many doctors believe that a fifty percent reduction in pain indicates a positive screening test.

Where can I get more information about APT?

Call the Medtronic Helpline at (800) 664-5111. ext. 855 to request a packet of information about APT Intrathecal and APT Neurostimulation or go to www.Medtronic.com.

Frequently Asked Questions About Advanced Pain Therapy Intrathecal

What is APT Intrathecal and how does it work?

APT Intrathecal uses a small pump that is surgically placed under the skin of the abdomen to deliver morphine directly to the intrathecal space, the fluid around the spinal cord. The medication is delivered through a small tube called a catheter that is also surgically placed. The spinal cord is like a highway for pain signals on their way to the brain, where the feeling of pain is experienced by your body. Because the drug is delivered directly to the spinal cord, where pain signals travel, APT Intrathecal can offer dramatic pain control, with a tiny fraction of the dose that would be required with pills. This helps minimize side effects.

How does the pump work?

The SynchroMed Infusion System has two parts that are both placed in the body during a surgical procedure: the catheter and the pump. The catheter is a small, soft tube. One end is connected to the pump, and the other is placed in the intrathecal space, where fluid flows around the spinal cord.

The pump is a round metal device that stores and releases prescribed amounts of medication directly into the intrathecal space. It is about one inch, 2.5 cm thick, three inches, 8.5 cm in diameter, and weighs about six ounces, 205 g. It is made of titanium, a light-weight, medical-grade metal.

The reservoir is the space inside the pump that holds the medication.

The fill port is a raised center portion of the pump through which the pump is refilled. Your doctor or nurse inserts a needle through your skin and through the fill port to fill the pump.

Some pumps have a side catheter access port that allows your doctor to inject other medications or sterile solutions directly in the catheter, bypassing the pump.

Is this a new therapy?

No. The SynchroMed System has been in use since 1988. It became commercially available in the U.S. for use with morphine to treat chronic pain in 1991. It has been used by thousands of patients worldwide.

How does Intrathecal medication work differently than oral medication?

APT Intrathecal delivers medication directly to the spinal cord, where pain signals are transmitted. In contrast, medications taken orally will have a systemic effect—they "flood" the whole body rather than staying concentrated in any single area. This often causes side effects such as sleepiness and confusion. These side effects may prevent your doctor from prescribing greater amounts of pain medication.

Will APT Intrathecal completely eliminate my pain?

While it may not be possible to completely eliminate your pain, APT Intrathecal may help you control it so your are more comfortable. Your doctor may prescribe additional oral medication, to relieve pain which occasionally "breaks through" the treatment.

Can I stop taking other pain medications with my pump?

Your doctor will determine whether you still need to take other medications. To prevent any negative side effects, do not make any changes in your current medication unless your doctor had directed you to do so.

What risks are associated with APT Intrathecal?

Any pain treatment can cause side effects. Talk with your doctor about side effects associated with APT Intrathecal. For example, because the pump and catheter are surgically placed, infections are possible. Other potential complications include fluid accumulation around the pump, spinal fluid leaks resulting in headache or other problems, and damage to the spinal cord. The catheter could become dislodged or blocked, or in rare cases, the pump could become dislodged or blocked, or could stop working. This could cause a reduction in or loss of pain relief and may require surgery to correct. Drug-related side effects can occur. They may include sleepiness, constipation, and upset stomach or vomiting. It is important that you discuss with your physician the potential risks, complications, and benefits about this therapy prior to giving your informed consent for treatment. Your doctor will be able to answer any questions you may have.

Will my pump be noticeable?
Depending on your size and shape, the pump will likely not be noticeable under regular clothes.

Will my insurance company pay for APT Intrathecal?
The system is approved by Medicare and many insurance carriers will pay for APT Intrathecal. However, as with many therapies, your doctor will have to get approval from your insurance company before you can receive APT Intrathecal. Consult your doctor or insurance carrier for more specific information.

What happens if the pump runs out of medication?
If the pump runs out of medication, your pain will return and you may experience withdrawal symptoms. Your doctor or nurse can tell when the pump will run out of medication by checking the pump with the programmer during your regular refill appointment. He or she will schedule a refill appointment for you before the pump runs out of medication. Make sure you write the date on your calendar and keep the scheduled refill appointment. In the event that you forget the date, the pump has an alarm to let you know when it is running out of medication. The pump emits a soft, high-pitched beeping sound repeated several times per minute. It is important to have your pump refilled before the alarm sounds. If you hear the alarm sound, call you doctor for an immediate refill appointment. Some people are unable to hear the alarm, so it is important to notify your doctor if you notice a change in pain relief or other changes.

How long will the pump last?
The battery that powers the pump will last three to five years, depending on the amount of medication it delivers.

How will I know when the pump needs to be replaced?
Your doctor or nurse will be able to tell you the state of the battery when he or she checks the pump with the programmer

during your regular refill appointment. In addition, the battery in the pump has a built-in alarm to let you know when the battery needs to be replaced. The pump emits a soft, high pitched beeping sound repeated several times per minute. If you hear the alarm sound, call your doctor immediately. Some people are unable to hear the alarm, so it is important to notify your doctor if you notice a change in pain relief or other changes.

What happens when the pump needs to be replaced?
Your doctor will arrange for the pump to be replaced at the end of the battery life. The catheter does not usually need to be replaced at this time.

Will the pump prevent me from traveling?
The pump will not prevent you from traveling as much as you're able, but be sure to schedule and keep all refill appointments. If you plan to travel far from home for long periods of time, notify your clinic. Your doctor will tell you about any prescription adjustments needed and work with you to coordinate any care or refills needed during your trip.

Will flying affect the pump?
Flying in commercial airlines will not generally affect the pump. However, talk to your doctor before long flights or flights in non-pressurized aircraft.

Will the pump set off the metal detector at the airport? How about theft detectors?
It might. You will receive an ID card that you can present to security personnel for clearance if necessary.

Will I be able to take hot baths or showers? Are saunas and hot tubs OKAY when I have a pump?
Most of the time, a hot bath, shower, sauna, or hot tub will not interfere with the pump's operation. However, you should talk with your doctor about other activities that may greatly affect the temperature or pressure of the pump, such as deep

heat therapy (diathermy), hyperbaric chamber treatment, or scuba diving.

Can I have an MRI with the pump? How about X-rays, radiation therapy, or diathermy?

MRI, X-rays, radiation therapy and diathermy may affect the function of the pump. Consult with your doctor before scheduling any additional therapies or diagnostic tests. Your doctor will determine if you need to take any precautions.

Can I use other magnetic devices with the pump?

Medtronic does not recommend using magnetic devices. A magnetic field, depending on the strength, could stop the pump.

What safety precautions should I follow with APT Intrathecal?

With APT Intrathecal, you can safely use most common household appliances, including microwave ovens, televisions, am/fm radios, stereos, remote controls, and video games.

CHAPTER TWENTY-ONE

How will my Doctor Know if I Can Benefit?

"I am grateful for understanding. It's the best thing in the world."
- Unknown

People with chronic, intractable pain often require a series of treatments from a team of health care professionals including your family doctor, other specialized doctors, nurses, physical therapists, occupational therapists, and psychologists.

When non-invasive treatments or surgery fail to provide pain relief, Medtronic Advanced Pain Therapies such as APT Neurostimulation or APT Intrathecal may be useful. Both therapies are non-destructive and reversible.

Your doctor, or a doctor to whom you are referred, will know whether these treatments may benefit you by going through a selection process. You may be a candidate for APT if:

* noninvasive treatments have failed
* corrective surgery would not help your pain
* you have no untreated chemical dependency problems
* routine psychological testing has been done
* you have no infections
* you are not allergic to any of the drugs used in the pump
* you have successfully completed a screening test

The screening test can help predict whether your pain can be relieved with APT. The screening test for APT Neurostimulation involves applying mild electrical stimulation to the spinal cord. The screening test for APT Intrathecal involves giving a dose of intrathecal morphine.

What to expect from your visit to the doctor:

Examination
Your doctor will do a thorough medical history and examination. Using this information, your doctor can assess whether you may be a candidate for Advanced Pain Therapy.

Psychological testing
People with chronic pain, their family members and significant others bring a unique mix of feelings, expectations, beliefs, personality traits, experiences, support systems, and skills to their pain treatment.

Because chronic pain involves both your body and mind, many doctors have people visit with a psychiatrist to determine if there are any psychological aspects of the pain that need to be treated. This is part of the process to ensure that you are an appropriate candidate for the therapy.

Advanced Pain Therapy Screening Tests
For both APT Neurostimulation and Apt Intrathecal, your doctor can do a screening test to help predict whether the therapy will relieve your pain. Many doctors believe that a fifty percent reduction in pain indicates a positive screening test.

Advanced Pain Therapy Neurostimulation Screening Test
Testing for APT Neurostimulation can be done as an outpatient procedure, or you may be admitted for a short hospital stay. The test procedure requires that you respond to certain sensations by letting your doctor know what you feel and where you feel it. Most people who experience a successful screening test can expect good to excellent pain relief when the system is surgically placed.

The process:

*   You receive local anesthesia, and then the doctor carefully inserts the lead, a special medical wire,   through a needle in the mid-back.

*   The doctor connects the lead wires to an external screener that allows the nurse or doctor to adjust   stimulation.

*   During the screening test, the doctor or nurse asks questions about the location and intensity of the   stimulation, or tingling sensation. This process   continues until they have found the best pain coverage.

*   After the lead is inserted, the test period may continue for several days. The screener, which is still attached   to the implanted lead, is sent home with you. During   this time, you test the system by adjusting the screener   to meet your pain management needs.

Advanced Pain Therapy Intrathecal Screening Test

Testing for APT Intrathecal can be done as an outpatient procedure, or you may be admitted for a short hospital stay. Your doctor will closely monitor your response to the pain medication given in this test and work with you to determine if you are a candidate for longterm therapy. One of two standard procedures is usually used to determine whether you experience significant, (at least fifty percent), pain relief:

* Bolus Injections. This procedure uses either a single injection or several injections of a small amount of pain medication into the intrathecal space, where fluid flows around the spinal cord.

* Continuous Infusion. This procedure uses a continuous infusion of pain medication that is delivered using a temporary catheter placed in the intrathecal or epidural   space and attached to an external pump. You may stay in   the hospital, or you may return home with the external   pump for several days or weeks. This test method is more   similar to the therapy delivered by the SynchroMed   Infusion system.

Advanced Pain Therapies & Your Responsibilities

There are general responsibilities you will have with APT, including:

* Keeping all scheduled appointments during treatment
* Asking questions about anything you do not understand
* Working together with your health care team to find the right levels of therapy to relieve your pain.
 * Following your doctor's directions
* Taking good care of yourself
* Reporting changes in pain levels, side effects, etc.

There are also specific responsibilities for each of the therapies...

Advanced Pain Therapy Intrathecal

* Schedule regular appointments with your doctor to refill your pump.

* Avoid physical activities that might involve the risk of trauma or a blow to the pump site.

* Watch for any unusual reaction to the specific medication you are receiving. Call your doctor if you have any unfamiliar or adverse side effects.

* Avoid alcohol and mood-altering drugs—they can cause serious side effects.

* Tell your family doctor and dentist you have a pump so they will be aware of this during any medical treatment.

* Tell family members and friends you have a pump so they will be aware of this during any medical treatment.

* If you plan to travel extensively, tell your doctor in advance to arrange for refills of the pump.

Advanced Pain Therapy Neurostimulation

* For six to eight weeks after the system is surgically placed, it is important to avoid bending, twisting, stretching or lifting objects over five pounds. This allows time for scar tissue to form and anchor the lead.

* Talk to your doctor before beginning any strenuous activity.

* Reduce the risk of damaging the Neurostimulation system by avoiding certain medical procedures, for example, magnetic resonance imaging, MRI. You may also want to take special precautions with electronic systems and   items

that use or generate magnetic fields; for example,   theft and
security detectors found in libraries and airports.

CHAPTER TWENTY-TWO

Medtronic Helpline

For further information about Advanced Pain Therapy Intrathecal and Neurostimulation, in the United States, call the Medtronic Helpline at: 1-800-664-5111, ext.855 to request a packet of information about APT Intrathecal and APT Neurostimulation or go to the website at: www.Medtronic.com.

Europe / Canada
(include. Eastern Europe)Medtronic of Canada Ltd.
Medtronic Europe S. A.6733 Kitimat Road
Route du Molliau Mississauga, Ontario L5N 1W3
CH-1131 Tolochenaz Canada
Switzerland Telephone: (905) 826-6620
Telephone: (41 21) 802 7000FAX: (905) 826-6620
FAX: (41 21) 8802 7900 Toll-free: 1-800-268-5346

Australia/Austria (43-1) 72734
Medtronic Australasia Pty. Ltd Denmark (45-45) 823 366
50 Strathallen Avenue Belgium (32-2) 4560900
Northbridge NSW 2063Finland (358-9) 134 511

Australia/France (33-1) 47146000
Telephone: (612) 9958 2999Italy (39-2) 661641
FAX: (612) 9958 7077Norway (47-67) 580680

Sweden (46-8) 583 593 00
The Netherlands (31-40) 2333888

United Kingdom (44-1923) 212213
Spain (34-1) 7355600
Germany (49-211) 52 93-0
Switzerland (41) 802 70

NOTE TO MY READERS:

Just saying:

Hello to my readers and fans. It is my hope that you have enjoyed my book, *Living Well With Chronic Pain* and that it has made a positive difference in your life.

Please share your love for *Living Well With Chronic Pain!* Those living with chronic pain tend to isolate themselves and I want to show them that they can have a normal life. And word–of-mouth is vital for an author to succeed. If you enjoyed the book, please leave a review at www.Amazon.com even if it's a sentence or two. That's how other readers find my books! Your reviews make a ton of difference and are so appreciated.

For an update on my other books and to be the first to hear about my *Sweet Home Colorado* series and all of my Colorado quirky, fun books, please take the time to sign up for my newsletter at www.judewillhoff.com (Note: Your email will never be shared and you can unsubscribe at anytime.)

The first book in my *Sweet Home Colorado* series is about a woman whose world is turned upside down because of her chronic pain. I have dedicated the book, *No Direction Home*, to those people living in the world who have to deal with chronic pain on a daily basis. If you are a chronic pain patient you are not alone. We're all in this together. Bless you on your journey.

~ Jude Willhoff

BUY A BOOK

You may purchase *Living Well With Chronic Pain* or Book One of the *Sweet Home Colorado* series called *No Direction Home*, Book Two, *Fly Away Home* and Book Three *Home Sweet Home* at

www.Amazon.com or at www.judewillhoff.com

~ Thank you!

Also, feel free to email me at jude2@prodigy.net I always answer each and every email—unless you're spamming me (lol!).

You can connect and hang with me in and on the following places:

Website: http://www.judewillhoff.com

Facebook: http://www.facebook.com/judewillhoff

Twitter: http://www.twitter.com/JudeWillhoff@JudeWillhoff

ABOUT THE AUTHOR

Jude Willhoff is a bestselling and award-winning author in both romance and nonfiction genres. *Living Well With Chronic Pain* was written as a book of her heart because she has Aracknoiditis and a spinal cord implant and lives with chronic pain. She wants to help people living with this disease by letting them know that with pain management they can live well with their ongoing condition. This book, *Living Well With Chronic Pain* is dedicated to those suffering with chronic pain.

Jude is an avid reader and a believer in all things romance. By day, she works alongside her husband with their real estate investments. "Though I could always use more time to write, the hours spent working with real estate are never dull and are a constant source of ideas for plots and characters." By night, she writes her contemporary romance and nonfiction books.

To celebrate Jude's official launch of *Living Well With Chronic Pain* she has happily included the first chapter of Book One of her *Sweet Home Colorado* series, *No Direction Home* for your enjoyment. Bless all of you who have chronic pain and may you have more manageable pain free days.

Thank you,
Jude Willhoff

~ SWEET HOME COLORADO ~
BOOK ONE

NO DIRECTION HOME

IT WAS AN OFFER SHE COULDN'T REFUSE...

Grace Sanders lost everything that mattered to her, her health to a debilitating disease and her husband to another woman. Experimental surgery gave her back her health, but couldn't repair her heart. Only time will heal the damage left behind by an unfaithful man so Grace throws herself into a new project—to save her trusting grandmother from being preyed on by an ex-con

FROM A MAN SHE COULDN'T TRUST...

Convicted of a crime he didn't commit, Seth Taylor lost everything that mattered to him, years with his daughter and the belief he'll never love again. Released from prison, he finds a job as a ranch foreman at the Cactus Rose Ranch in Cedar Falls, Colorado. His widowed boss refuses to let growing old destroy her dreams and she believes in second chances.

Second chances are what both Grace and Seth need to create their own Sweet Home Colorado.

PREVIEW OF BOOK ONE

~ *Sweet Home Colorado Series* ~

No Direction Home

Chapter One

Being stranded in the high mountains of Colorado with a blizzard on the way wasn't what Grace Sanders had set out to do. Low clouds wrapped wispy gray fingers around her car while the tree-covered mountainside disappeared into the gloom.

The eerie red glow from her emergency flashers illuminated the interior of the car. With a groan she lifted her head from the steering wheel and stared out the windshield.

Anxious to get to the Cactus Rose Ranch, she punched in the roadside assistance number for the umpteenth time praying for a signal. *Nothing. Damn. Enough of this pity poor me crap.* She pushed the car door open.

Icy mist soaked her thin silk dress, making her teeth chatter. California wear wasn't suited to the frigid mountain temperatures. She knew better, but getting home to protect her Nana from that smooth talking cowboy had been the only thing on her mind. As far as she was concerned all men were pigs.

Making love to you is like screwing a corpse. Even after all this time, the memory of her ex-husband Lee's parting words still had the ability to wound. He'd betrayed her, ripped a hole in her heart the size of Montana. She pushed the unwanted recollection to the far corners of her mind and shivered.

Her bare skin prickled with goose bumps against the chill as the trunk popped open and she pulled out the heavy lug wrench. With a sick taste of fear settling in the pit of her stomach, she stared at the spare tire bolted to the trunk floor.

Could she lift it? Her spinal cord implant was working, but she couldn't risk pulling lose any of the fine wires traveling up her spine and into her central nervous system. How much did a tire weigh? The doctors had said not to lift anything over ten pounds. What to do? Lord, she hated feeling helpless.

She unbolted the tire and tugged at it. An instant strain started up her lower back and she had to let go. "Damn." She moved around the car and kicked the flat tire with a vengeance.

From out of the dense fog, a semi barreled past and sprayed her with cold dirty water. Brushing grit and hot tears from her face, she kicked the tire once again, only hurting her toe. "Damn, damn, damn." She raised her foot to strike it a third time.

"Whoa, little lady, what'd that tire do to you?"

Grace jumped at the sound of a deep voice coming from behind her. She was no longer alone. Her heart beat an unsteady rhythm against her ribcage as she turned. A stranger stood five feet away in the dusky light smiling at her with a twinkle in his eyes. At least he was smiling. Maybe he wasn't a serial killer.

"Where'd you come from?" Frustration quivered in her voice as she tried to sound in complete control of the situation.

He had materialized in the dreary, misty evening without a sound. Grace brushed dripping water from her face while he glanced at the ruined tire.

"Ma'am." His fingers touched the brim of his Stetson. "I was heading back to the ranch and saw your flashing lights. Thought you might be having some kind of trouble."

Living in LA, she had learned to be cautious with strangers. However, she couldn't change the tire by herself and the rugged cowboy did seem harmless. She detested admitting defeat, but in this situation she had no choice. "I can't get the tire out of the trunk." Through the swirling fog she could make out the dim lights of a house sitting high on a hill in the distance. A horse nickered. Grace glanced at the large brown animal with a splash of white on its head. It stood tied to a fence post next to the road. Apparently, Mr. Cowboy was telling the truth.

"Ma'am, I'd be happy to oblige." Feather-like laugh lines crinkled around his deep blue eyes.

He probably thought she was nuts. No doubt a dripping wet overweight blond kicking a tire in the icy rain, must make quite a picture. No matter how embarrassed she was, she needed his strength. *One more time this damn disease wins.* Shivering, she folded her arms across her chest and nodded. "Okay."

"You're freezing." He took off his rain slicker and placed it around her damp shoulders. "Put this on while I help you get back on the road." He tugged the coat snug to her body. When his fingertips accidently grazed her neck she felt his warmth pass to her skin.

"Thanks," she mumbled. Enveloped in the large coat she watched him work. It had been a long time since anyone besides the doctors had touched her. The aroma of leather and man rose from the coat and tickled her nose. He easily removed the tire and the rest of the tools from the trunk as if they weighed nothing.

To her surprise, he took off his shirt and wrapped it around the tire iron. She swallowed a gasp. Self-conscious about her reaction she clutched the coat close. After working on movie sets in Hollywood for the past several years, she wasn't naive, but this man made her feel things that she thought were long behind her. The sight of him made her want things she couldn't have. She had never felt this kind of instant attraction, not even with Lee.

A smile crossed his face as he gazed up at her. "The dry shirt helps me to get a better grip." He loosened the bolts with each tug of the wrench.

Fascinated, she watched the misty rain drip off his sinewy muscles, down his back and over a washboard stomach with dark chest hair curling in tiny ringlets. He tossed the bolts into the upturned hubcap.

His blue eyes flashed in friendship when he glanced in her direction. She wasn't a prude, but she was glad it was getting darker, not wanting him to see the blush on her cheeks. It had been a long time since she'd seen a handsome man shirtless. Though her heart lifted at the sight, she had no business staring at him. Those days were behind her.

He slipped the ruined tire free. "Looks like you ran over something that punched a hole in it." He nodded toward the damaged tire and laid it on the ground. Placing the spare on the wheel, he tightened down the bolts and shrugged on his damp shirt. "There you go. It should get you where you're going." He hit the hubcap into place with the palm of his hand and tossed the flat in the trunk next to her luggage.

When he slammed it shut, she saw him glance at her LA Lady vanity plates. He didn't say anything. Aware of her soggy, deflated appearance in contrast to her sensuous thoughts she handed him his coat. "You've been a godsend."

"Glad I could help." He held the car door open so she could slide behind the wheel. After putting his slicker on, he nodded toward the sky. "This storm is going to get worse. It's best you get on your way to somewhere dry."

Grace was glad to be back in the warm car. "You're right. Thanks a lot." He didn't know how right he was. The last thing she needed with her chronic condition was to get sick. She flipped on the headlights and waved at the stranger as she drove back onto the road heading home to the Cactus Rose Ranch. In just a short time she'd be home.

Warm air flowed through the car as she glanced into the rearview mirror and brushed her hair back with her fingertips. Thanks to that handsome cowboy, she would dry out and make it home. Still chilled, she turned the heat on high.

She'd been in terrible pain before the surgery and unable to walk. Being dependant on other people had been the hardest thing she had ever dealt with in her life. Through hard work and sheer determination, she had regained her independence. In her heart, Grace knew coming home to the ranch to help her grandmother was the best thing.

Over the years, she'd made solo trips home and had brought Nana and Papa to Los Angeles for visits but it hadn't been nearly enough. She should've done more.

Many miles later and now dry, she finally turned onto the two mile drive to the Cactus Rose Ranch. Right on cue, big fat snowflakes gently swirled in the headlights. She loved snow and hadn't seen it for years. This was a good omen.

In the distance, the lights shone bright through the windows of the two-story log home nestled among the large rocks and blue spruce trees on the hillside. There was a time she didn't think she'd ever see this place again.

Home. A nostalgia she hadn't expected tugged her lips into a smile just before a mind-numbing pain shot down her right leg. Scary-down-to-the-core-of-her-being pain. Pain that would never go away. Grimacing, she pulled into the circular driveway next to the house. *Not now.* She took several deep breaths and willed the fire burning down her leg to become more bearable. With the pain toned down to tolerable, she rushed from the car toward her Nana's loving arms.

Her small white-haired grandmother hurried through the thickening snowflakes to greet her with a wide grin on her weathered face. "Gracie Bell, for goodness sake, when you said you'd be on your way I didn't think you meant this soon."

Gracie Bell. She hadn't heard that endearment for such a long time it caused a lump to lodge in her throat. She swallowed it down. "I wanted to surprise you. I left the hospital as soon as I could." And when Grace had found out a strange man was running the ranch she didn't have much choice.

"Well, whatever, it was worth it to get you home. Are you okay?" She held her at arm's length for a moment, then hugged her tight again.

"I had a flat, but I'm okay, just a little tired. Nana, I'm home. I'm really home," she murmured against the familiar shoulder, inhaling her grandma's fragrance mingled with the scent of snow. Her heart pounded with joy. The Cactus Rose Ranch had been her home since the age of five, after her parents died in an auto accident.

"Yes, you are. Come inside. We'll get your things later." She wrapped an arm around Grace's waist as they walked up the steps, across the wide country porch and into the comfortable living room.

The pungent smell of wood burning in the fireplace floated through the air. The brown leather sofa piled high with soft mauve and green flowered pillows, beckoned to Grace. Tired and needing to sit for a moment, she sank into its welcome softness.

"Tell me, how was your trip? Has it completely worn you out?" Nana's full head of thick curly white hair glistened in the soft light. Her warm brown eyes showed concern.

"No, I took my time and I'm doing fine. I'm tired from driving, but nothing more." She wasn't about to worry Nana with her problems. She just couldn't tell her about the stream of fire burning through her body. She glanced around the room at family pictures and well-worn comfortable furniture. It hadn't changed much. Ollie, Nana's orange and white cat, snoozed peacefully in her recliner. He had been around for about eighteen years, a fixture in the home, sleeping on any lap that would take him.

Grace laid her head back against the sofa taking slow deep breaths and adjusted to take weight off her spine. "How's Ollie? He looks the same."

"Like me, slowing down, old and cranky, but he's doing fine. Spoiled rotten." She smiled. "Are you hungry?"

"No. I ate in Grand Junction."

"I'll fix you a cup of hot tea. It'll help you relax." Nana rushed across the room and into the open kitchen.

Grace followed at a slower pace. "That does sound good, but you don't have to wait on me. I can do it myself."

"It's nothing, sweetie." Nana poured hot water over the tea bags waiting in the large coffee mugs. "Sit down. I know you're worn out." She pulled a cushioned chair from the oak table and gently pushed Grace into it.

The open kitchen was warm and inviting with the smell of fresh baked banana bread lingering in the air. "Something smells good." She enjoyed the aroma, knowing Nana had baked for her.

"Yes, I made your favorite." She pushed a steaming mug of cinnamon apple tea in front of Grace. "This will warm you up."

"Great." Looking out the wide wall of windows over the kitchen sink, Grace watched the snow falling silently to the ground. It was peaceful. She'd missed Nana and home.

"Were the roads bad?"

"No, not really, lots of rain, but no snow until I got here." Clasping cold fingers around the warm mug Grace sipped the tea.

"You've probably been a little ahead of the storm all the way. We've been preparing for it for the past few days. Seth already moved the cattle down to the lower pasture."

She tensed at the mention of Seth. She would have to tread lightly on this topic with Nana. "So things are working out with Seth?" Nana had hired the new foreman after Papa passed, but Grace had never met the man.

"Yes, real well. I don't know what I'd do without him. He's always ahead of the game. Seems to know by instinct when bad weather is coming. I've let him take over the bookkeeping for me. Other than your grandfather, he's the best foreman I've ever worked with."

Oh, my goodness. The man is in charge of the books? A twinge of apprehension tugged at the corners of Grace's mind. "Be careful. He's a stranger and there are a lot of crooks in the world—men who wouldn't balk at taking advantage of a widow owning a spread like this." After all, she had loved Lee and look what he had done to her. When the going got rough, he left her high and dry. "He might be after something."

Nana laughed. "Nonsense. Wait till you meet him. He should be home anytime now. He and a few of the ranch hands were up north helping out the Wilsons. Jim Wilson broke his leg and Sally has had her hands full." She took a bite of bread before she continued. "By the way, he stays upstairs. It was a shame to have all those bedrooms sitting there collecting dust." She grinned. "I hated living in this big old house rambling around by myself." She busied herself wiping nonexistent crumbs from the table and avoided Grace's shocked gaze.

"You've moved him into the house?" Grace's voice cracked with emotion when she set her cup down with a clatter. "What were you thinking?" She frowned. "What's wrong with him staying in the bunk house with the rest of the hired help?"

"Nothing." Nana stopped fidgeting and gave her a direct gaze—one filled with strong conviction. "When I came down with pneumonia last year, he moved in to take care of me. He helped me with a lot of things when I was sick and I happen to like his company."

"You didn't tell me you were sick." Once again, Grace hadn't been able to be there for her grandmother. Guilt slammed into her.

"You had enough on your plate. There was no need to worry you." Nana pursed her lips and sat back casually in the chair, looking like she had when she'd reassured Grace about her new second grade teacher. "I know you'll get along with him. You'll see."

Fatigue from the long trip washed over Grace as she gripped the edge of the table. "Okay, I'll take your word for it."

A complete stranger was living down the hall from her naive grandmother. During Grace's confinement in the nursing home, the back surgery and rehabilitation, the man had worked his way into Nana's heart and home.

Why would a man move in with an old lady if he didn't have ulterior motives? Maybe he was one of those types who married widows to get their life savings. Was he after the ranch, Nana's money, or both?

The homestead had been in the family for three generations. She couldn't stand by and let some kind of con artist cheat Nana out of it. Simply put, Grace couldn't keep her mouth shut. "Did you have the guy checked out?"

Nana rolled her eyes. "There you go, again."

"Where's he from? Does he have any family?"

"I know what you're asking and I'm telling you, I didn't have to do anything like that. I know a good person when I see one and Seth has a good heart. He's worked on ranches since he was a boy. Grew up in Texas. He has family back there and gets letters but throws them in the trash. Those folks must've hurt him real bad for him to do something like that."

She sighed and didn't want to argue with Nana on her first night home. "I hope you know what you're doing." She bit her tongue and shut up. After the experience with her ex, Grace couldn't see much good in any man but this wasn't the time to continue the conversation.

Until now, the possibility had never occurred to her that Nana might still be attracted to men or need some kind of companionship other than the cat. Yet, Nana was sharp and energetic for her years. Confusing thoughts raced around Grace's head while she wondered if Nana had dated anyone over the past few years. She hadn't mentioned anything.

Grace sighed. She just wasn't up to dealing with this tonight. At the moment, everything hurt. Feeling ancient, she tried to hide a yawn.

"Dear, you're falling asleep on your feet. Why don't you take a hot bath and get comfortable? I'll call one of the boys from the bunk house to bring your luggage in from the car."

Grace allowed herself to be manipulated by Nana's smooth shift in conversation. "A hot shower sounds like heaven. I think I will. I've been cold all day." She walked over to hug Nana. "Have you lost weight?" She could feel Nana's small-boned body through her heavy sweater.

"Maybe a few pounds. I was getting too heavy." Nana laughed and walked with Grace out of the kitchen.

"That'll be the day." Taking a closer look at Nana, she noticed the frailties and dark circles under her eyes. Her liveliness was still there, but Nana was in her sixties. She had always been in good health, but she didn't look quite right. "When I'm finished I'll come back down for another cup of tea."

"Okay, I'll keep the water on." Nana walked into the living room and Grace watched her click on the TV to the evening news and settle back into the recliner as Ollie jumped onto her lap. Worry tugged at the corner of her mind. Would Nana tell her if something was wrong?

Maybe not, though Grace fully intended to worm it out of her. However, not tonight. Stifling another yawn, she turned down the hall. She rubbed the well worn oak railing as she climbed the stairs to her room, remembering the many times she and her best friend Cindy had slid down the banister.

Going into the bedroom was like taking a step back in time. Sitting on the bed for a minute to relax she looked around at the things she had left behind. The same antique white lace curtains hung over the wide windows. Her favorite forest green throw lay across the foot of the double bed.

Sighing, she got up and grabbed her robe that still hung on the back of the adjoining bathroom door. She turned on the welcoming spray and adjusted the water temperature.

A few moments later, she dropped clothing to the floor and stepped into the warmth. Letting the hot water trickle over tight muscles, it slowly took away some of the bone-tired fatigue and began to ease her pain. She would sleep well tonight, but first she would visit with Nana. The last thing she wanted was for her grandmother to be upset about their disagreement over Seth.

Coming out of the shower, she wrapped herself in a huge fluffy towel. She dried off and pulled her soft blue robe against her bare skin. It was thin and a little small since she'd put on a few pounds, but it would keep the chill away until she could find some pajamas.

She picked up a comb and ran it through damp hair and worked the knots out of the long strands. The woman staring back from the mirror was a stranger. She wasn't the same person she used to be. She had gained thirty pounds after going through the divorce and surgery. The stubborn chin, brown eyes and long natural dark blond hair were the same but the person inside was someone else, someone she was discovering with each new day.

With hair dry and body refreshed from the shower, Grace began to feel human again. A loud thump sounded outside the bedroom door. She froze. *Oh God. Had Nana fallen?* In a panic, she rushed out the door and flew around the corner straight into a solid chest. A man's chest.

Strong arms wrapped around her nearly naked body as she noticed luggage strewn around the floor. The smell of man, horse and leather tickled her nose. Startled, she glanced up to see familiar blue eyes staring back at her. *The sexy cowboy.* For an instant, being held in his arms, all her loneliness welded together in one upsurge of yearning. Grace's heart thumped dangerously as a warm glow flowed through her.

She stepped back and clutched the skimpy robe together, knowing that it didn't leave much to the imagination. It was hard to be coherent when she was this close to him. He stood there with a slow bemused grin lifting the corner of his mouth. "You? What are you doing here?" she asked.

He touched the tip of his fingers to the brim of his hat. "Hello, ma'am, I'm Seth Taylor. I live here." His voice swept over her like a blanket fresh from a warm dryer. Soft and smooth. The grin spread across his face as he gave her the once over. "Well, if it isn't the LA Lady. So you're Nana's granddaughter. She told me about you." His eyes lit up like he could see right through her robe.

His nearness was disturbing and exciting. She struggled to get her traitorous thoughts under control. "Yes...you'll have to forgive me. I...I didn't expect to see you outside my bedroom door." Flustered, she pushed a strand of hair out of her face. She was babbling, and naked beneath the flimsy robe. She felt her nipples harden from the chill in the hallway.

Embarrassed on so many levels, she resolved the first thing she was going to do was change those damned vanity plates. She'd hated them since Lee had given them to her for a birthday present. They were pretentious. Seth must think she was a California flake. What had Nana told him?

His eyes lit with a mischievous glint. "I'm sorry. I didn't mean to startle you. I was dropping off your luggage before I went to my room." He leaned down and picked up the overturned suitcases and set them inside her door. "It's been a long day and I'm sure you're tired." Nervous in his steady gaze, she couldn't speak. "We'll talk more in the morning." He smiled. "Evening, ma'am." He touched the brim of his hat again, turned and walked down the hall.

Her stomach churned with anxiety and frustration as she stood in the familiar hallway, rooted to the spot. Her fingers still clutched the top of her robe, but she couldn't control the slight trembling within her. The man who had changed her tire was Seth—the cowboy Nana had hired. He wasn't what she had expected. Somehow, she thought he would be older.

Holding her raw emotion in check she breathed in shallow quick gasps. Why, he was about her age, thirty-six or so—but with a strong healthy body, full of virility. The man oozed sex appeal and damn she was attracted to him.

If he looked this good after a long day of hard work, she couldn't begin to imagine what he would look like when he was fresh from the shower. No, she shouldn't go there, but there was no denying it. The man was drop-dead gorgeous. With that shaggy mustache and his brown wavy hair peeking out from under the Stetson, even tinged with a bit of silver at his temples, he looked—tempting. And those magnetic blue eyes. Geez.... He definitely made her heart race. *Please, God, have mercy. Let him be bald under that hat.*

No wonder Nana was taken with him. All that charm in one package was hard to handle. *Life just isn't fair.*

She blinked and curled her toes against the plush beige carpet. What was wrong with her? After Lee, she didn't think she'd ever want to be with another man, and out of nowhere, here were all these feelings she thought were long dead. This was crazy. She was losing her grip—this was the man who was up to no good.

"Christ, Grace, snap out of it. One good-looking cowboy and you're drooling. Get a hold of yourself." She muttered under her breath as she pulled a flannel nightgown and another robe from her suitcase and redressed. Sighing, she headed down the stairs. "For heaven's sake, he's just a man." And she'd sworn off men altogether.

Nana looked up from where she stood warming her hands by the crackling fire. "Grace, dear. There you are. Did the hot shower help?"

"Yes, I feel better." She hesitated for a second. "I met Seth. He's the man who changed my flat tire today." She struggled with mixed emotions as she sat on the comfortable sofa and pulled her feet underneath the long robe. "I was surprised to see him, here in the house."

"It must be fate that you met earlier." Nana laughed. "I knew you'd hit it off."

She was too tired to disagree. Besides, the man had been nice enough to help her out of a fix with the flat tire. Maybe she was making mountains out of molehills. She smiled, knowing Nana was amused by the coincidence. Regardless, deep inside, being home touched her heart and other than being around Seth, she felt at ease for the first time in a long time.

"Honey, I can't begin to tell you how happy I am you're here to stay. I've missed you so much."

Nana sat in the recliner and Ollie crawled into her lap. He purred audibly as he rubbed his head against her hand. She scratched him under the chin, causing his purr to rise in volume. "Ollie is glad you're home, too."

"Oh yeah, he's thrilled to see me." Grace chuckled softly

and gazed around the room. A picture of her parents sat on the right side of the mantel. Nana and Papa were on the left and long-ago snapshots of her growing up dominated the rest of the mantel between the green plants and gold candlesticks. With these pictures and Nana's penchant for chatting, it dawned on her, Seth must already know more about her than Lee ever had, since Nana seemed to be taken with him and had hardly spoken to Grace's husband.

She guessed he hadn't recognized her on the road because of the weight she'd gained. That...and the fact she'd looked like a drowned mutt. But surely he had put two and two together when he'd seen the license plates. Why didn't he say something?

Outside, the snow continued to fall with the wind whistling around the back of the house. Grace glanced out the window toward the porch light. "It's really coming down. I hope it doesn't turn into a blizzard."

"No worries, the big storm missed us. Now we're only going to get a few inches. It's not going to amount to much." Nana continued to pet Ollie, pleasing the kitty immensely.

That reminded her.... "Nana, what are your plans for tomorrow? I need to go into town and do a few things. Would you like to go with me?" The hiss and pop of the wood fire relaxed Grace while she sat and watched the flames.

"Oh, I'm sorry, I can't. I volunteer at the hospital two days a week and tomorrow I work in the gift shop from ten to six. Maybe I can switch with someone."

"No, don't worry about it. I'm sure Cedar Falls hasn't changed that much." She stretched and yawned, thinking Nana must be okay if she worked at the hospital on a regular basis.

"No, it's about the same. We did get a new Safeway store and a strip mall over by the bank."

"Good. I have to do some shopping and get Colorado tags for my car." Grace ran a hand through her hair, holding out a long strand, looking at the splint ends. "And I need a haircut."

"Cindy's still on Main Street next to the post office. She seems to be doing well. Every time I go to get my hair done, the place is packed with customers." Nana put Ollie on the floor and walked over to the fireplace. "She always asks about you." Nana picked up the wrought iron poker. "Did you know she and her husband split up last year? He was running around on her with some woman in Denver." Flustered, Nana glanced away. "Oh, I'm sorry, honey. I shouldn't have said that."

Grace took a deep breath. It was ironic her and Cindy's marriages had suffered the same fate—betrayal. "It's okay. I'm over it." She picked lint off the flowered sofa pillow she held against her chest. "After I became ill, I couldn't be a real wife to Lee. And he couldn't handle it."

Shadows of past hurts marched through her mind like a funeral procession...back to years ago. At the height of her pain and suffering, she had caught him in the swimming pool with a naked woman. Worse, he hadn't even cared—he just laughed and returned to the woman's arms, leaving Grace broken and crushed both physically and emotionally. It was a hard lesson, but well learned. The marriage was over. The next day she let him move her into a nursing home, tossing her aside like yesterday's stale donuts.

Nana poked the log in the fireplace with a vengeance, bringing Grace back to the present. "A real wife? That's hogwash. The man was no good. You were going through a tough time. Instead of taking up with another woman at the first sign of trouble, he should've been there for you, stood by you."

Grace watched bright orange sparks fly up the chimney as Nana pushed the log around the grate. She suppressed hurt feelings under the appearance of indifference and chose her words carefully. "My life has changed. I've had to accept things as they are, not as I want them to be. When someone is in great pain like I was, you don't feel like making love. And let's face it, that's the backbone of any marriage." She hesitated. This was hard to talk about. "He didn't want to wait for me to get better."

"Sweetheart, there's a lot more to a relationship than sex." Nana poked the log angrily. "I'm going to tell you something about Lee. I should've told you years ago." She pushed her small round wire-rimmed glasses up on the bridge of her nose. "When you were living in Denver and engaged Papa saw Lee with another woman. He thought it was some kind of business

dinner or he would've told you and spared you this heartache."
She frowned and hit the log again. "You don't need him. There
will be someone else, someone better for you."

Grace stopped playing with her hair. This conversation was
inevitable. She might as well get it over with. "I know about
his affair with the woman in Denver. It came out when we
separated. Since she is an attorney, too, they have a lot in
common." She sighed deeply. "Actually, she lives in LA now
and they're together." The witch had been the woman in her
swimming pool.

Nana started toward the open kitchen. "Well, you're better
off without him. And this calls for something stronger than tea.
Would you like a glass of White Zinfandel?" She picked up
two long-stemmed wine glasses and a chilled bottle and headed
back to Grace.

"Sounds good to me." Grace sat up and took the wine glass.
"I've worked it out in my mind. I wish them well. I want Lee to
be happy." She tried to push down the fact it still hurt. "In his
own way, he was good to me. He was fair with the divorce."

"Of course he was fair. Humph...he had no choice. You
caught him in the act." Nana filled their glasses.

The wine was cool against Grace's throat. She didn't want
to talk about Lee anymore. "I want to put this behind me and
get on with what's left of my life." She sighed. "I need you to
understand that I have to protect myself. Stress of any kind
causes me to physically hurt more."

"Honey, I had no idea. I don't want you to hurt. What can I
do?"

"Nothing. It's all up to me. I have to let the emotional
baggage with Lee go. Then I can move on to better times. It's
too painful to remember." She ran a hand through her hair. "In
my own defense, I must wish him well. Now, do you
understand?"

"Yes, I think I do. And you're right, he isn't worth hurting
over." Nana sipped the wine. "I'm proud of you for the way
you've handled what's happened to you. But, like I said, one
day a good man will come into your life. He won't care about
your condition. He'll love you for being you."

Grace frowned and shook her head. "I've given up on the

idea of another man. I had a lot of time to think while I was in the rehab center. It's just me. No one else. And that's how it has to be." She set the glass on the coffee table. "I wouldn't want to burden anyone with my physical problems. I still might end up in a wheelchair. I couldn't put that responsibility on someone else." Grace focused blindly on the yellow-orange flames dancing high in the fireplace. A life alone. As much as she knew that was her future, she couldn't escape the emptiness inside.

"Honey, you can't think that way. They said you'd never walk again. Now look at you. You've come so far. You're a success story, an inspiration to other people who have this disease. You have to stay positive."

"It's okay. I am positive. I'm being realistic about my life. I'm thirty-six and have to face facts. I can't work as a make-up artist anymore. My career is over." She sighed. "I don't know what I'm going to do, but marriage is the last thing on my mind. I know I can't be a normal wife—a man doesn't want to tie himself to an invalid." She sighed.

"Anyway, I can live my life without a man and I'll find something else to do." Grace had to say these things to convince herself. It wasn't that she didn't want someone in her life. It was that physically she wasn't good enough to keep them happy. Plus she was considered one hundred percent disabled—that wasn't much to offer anyone.

Nana sat on the sofa beside her and held her hands. Moisture shimmered in her warm brown eyes when she squeezed Grace's fingers. "You know this will always be your home. You'll never have to worry about a place to live."

She gazed deep into Nana's eyes and saw the unconditional love shining back. She couldn't stay upset with her. "I know. Thank you...I...I love you." She lay down on the sofa, resting her head in Nana's lap like she had as a child.

Nana stroked a hand through Grace's hair. "You're bone tired and heart sick. You haven't had time to adjust to what's happened to you." She continued caressing her hair. "Rest, child. You'll find yourself."

Grace knew Nana would help her make things right. She snuggled against Nana. For the first time in ages, she felt safe and loved. She finally relaxed and felt on the verge of falling asleep.

"Sleep, baby, you're plumb worn out physically and emotionally." Nana sighed. "Love heals. One day soon, a good man will come into your life and he'll help you put all this behind you."

As Grace drifted off to sleep she thought she heard Nana murmur, "And I know just the man."

BUY A BOOK

You may purchase *Living Well With Chronic Pain* or Book One of the *Sweet Home Colorado* series called *No Direction Home*, Book Two, *Fly Away Home* and Book Three *Home Sweet Home* at

www.Amazon.com or at www.judewillhoff.com

~ Thank you!

5231199R00109

Printed in Great Britain
by Amazon.co.uk, Ltd.,
Marston Gate.